Busy Cookbook for 2

Includes 30 Quick & Light Dinner Recipes for You & Your Partner When You're Busy

by Olivia Rogers

Copyright © 2017 By Olivia Rogers
All rights reserved. No part of this book may be reproduced in any form without permission in writing from the author. No part of this publication may be reproduced or transmitted in any form or by any means, mechanic, electronic, photocopying, recording, by any storage or retrieval system, or transmitted by email without the permission in writing from the author and publisher.
For information regarding permissions write to author at Olivia@TheMenuAtHome.com
Reviewers may quote brief passages in review.

Please note that credit for the images used in this book go to the respective owners. You can view this at: TheMenuAtHome.com/image-list

Olivia Rogers
TheMenuAtHome.com

Table of Contents

Introduction — 6
Section 1: Light Appetizer Recipes — 7
1. Turkey and Lettuce Chinese Wraps — 7
2. Mini Almond Cheese Balls — 9
3. Bean Dip with Cannellini and Spinach — 11
4. BLT with Egg — 13
5. Chicken Empanadas — 15
6. Open-Faced Radish Sandwiches — 18
7. Light Microwave Chips — 20
8. Black Bean and Cheese Nachos — 22
9. Lentil and Carrot Soup — 24
Section 2: Healthy Meal Options — 26
10. Cauliflower Chicken — 26
11. Chicken Parmesan — 28
12. Sweet & Spicy Shrimp with Noodles — 30
13. Grilled Chicken with Salad and Pineapple Dressing — 32
14. Citrus Beef Kebabs — 34
15. Thai Prawns with Pineapple Rice — 36
16. Asparagus and Potato Frittatas — 38
17. Fish Stew — 40
18. Red Pepper Chicken — 42
19. Moroccan Veggie Stew — 44
20. Meatloaf — 46
Section 3: Sweet on The Tooth, Light on The Tummy — 48
21. Cheesecake Brownies — 48

22. Power Bars _____ 50

23. Chia Seed Yogurt _____ 52

24. Blueberry Cobbler _____ 53

25. Chocolate and Zucchini Bread _____ 55

Section 4: Energizing Healthy Beverages _____ 57

26. Pumpkin Smoothie _____ 57

27. Green Concoction _____ 59

28. Citrus Coconut Water _____ 60

29. Frappuccino _____ 61

30. Wasabi Tuna Kebabs _____ 62

31. Puff Pastry Pizza _____ 64

32. Garlic Chili Shrimp _____ 66

33. Tuna & White Bean Salad _____ 68

34. Summery Shrimp Salad _____ 70

35. Crispy Artichokes in Aged Balsamic _____ 72

36. Winter Squash Soup with Pumpkin Seeds _____ 74

37. Chili Made Easy _____ 76

38. Clam Chowder _____ 78

39. Simplified Cioppino _____ 80

40. Veggie & Almond Couscous _____ 82

41. Paella _____ 84

42. Tomato Bouillabaisse _____ 86

43. Orange Chicken Stir Fry _____ 88

44. Sausage & Kale Fettuccine _____ 90

45. Mushroom & Sausage Lasagna _____ 92

46. Sautéed Ham & Brussels Sprouts _____ 94

47. Salmon in Blueberry Sauce _____ 96

48. Chicken Masala _____ 98
49. Lamb Provencal _____ 100
50. Glazed Pork Chops _____ 102
Conclusion _____ 104
Final Words _____ 105
Disclaimer _____ 107

Introduction

Whether there's a potluck in an hour and you forgot to prepare a dish or you just came home from work and don't know what to make, use this cookbook to whip up delicious yet simple dishes to satisfy everyone.

Each recipe in this book is simple and fast without sacrificing any flavor. These dishes are deceptively easy while still creating expert flavor combinations that will convince people you spent hours in the kitchen tediously preparing this meal.

Lack of time is no longer an excuse to pass up on quality, delicious (and healthy) meals! Read through the recipes in this book and get inspired.

Section 1: Light Appetizer Recipes

1. Turkey and Lettuce Chinese Wraps

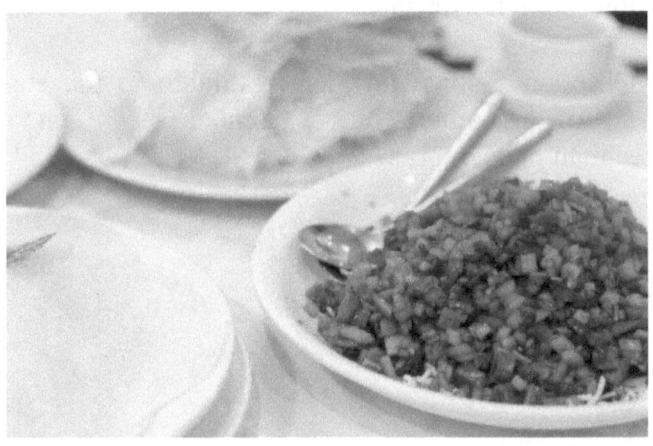

Preparation Time: 1 hour (including 30 minutes of active cooking)
Serving size: 2

Ingredients

- ½ red bell peppers (diced finely)
- ½ a carrot (shredded)
- 1 head of lettuce (separate the leaves)
- ½ 8oz can, water chestnuts (chopped and rinsed)
- ¼ cup of fresh chopped herbs (basil, mint, chives or cilantro)
- ½ tablespoon fresh ginger (minced)
- ½ pound lean turkey (ground)
- ¼ cup brown rice (instant)

- 1 teaspoon sesame oil

- ¼ cup chicken broth

- 1 tablespoon hoisin sauce

- ½ teaspoon 5-spice powder (available in the supermarket; blend of cinnamon, cloves, fennel seed, star anise and Szechuan peppercorns)

- ¼ teaspoon salt

- Water for boiling rice

Method

1. Boil water in a saucepan. Once, the water is boiled, add the rice, and cover the saucepan.

2. Cook for 5 minutes on low flame. Remove saucepan from flame once the rice has cooked.

3. Meanwhile, take a nonstick pan, put it over medium to high flame and add oil to it. Once the oil is heated, add ginger and ground turkey. Use a spoon (wooden) to crumble the turkey, till its cooked through (roughly about 6 minutes).

4. Then slowly stir and add the broth, 5-spice powder, salt, hoisin sauce, rice, bell peppers and water chestnuts. Cook for about a minute or till it is heated throughout.

5. Lay out the lettuce leaves on the plate (for serving), scoop some turkey mixture on to it, sprinkle herbs and carrots and roll the lettuce into wraps. Enjoy!

2. Mini Almond Cheese Balls

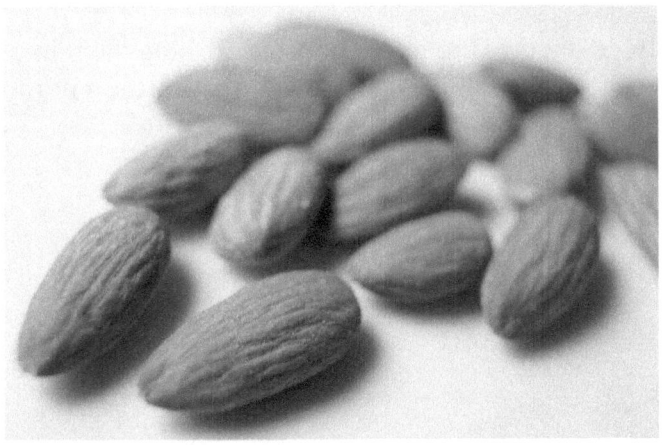

Preparation Time: 45 minutes
Serving size: 9 (of 2 balls each)

Ingredients

- 1 teaspoons honey
- 4 oz. goat cheese
- ½ teaspoon fresh thyme (minced)
- ¼ teaspoon lemon rind (grated)
- 1/4 cup chopped almonds (roasted and salted)
- 4 oz. plain almond milk cream cheese

Method

1. Beat both the cheeses, honey and lemon rind at a medium speed in a bowl for 2 minutes, until smooth) and freeze for 15 minutes.

2. Using a food processor, grind thyme and nuts into a fine mixture and lay it on to a dish.

3. Divide the mixture into 9 portions, rolling them into balls and freeze for 10 minutes. Roll each ball in the nut mixture and serve.

3. Bean Dip with Cannellini and Spinach

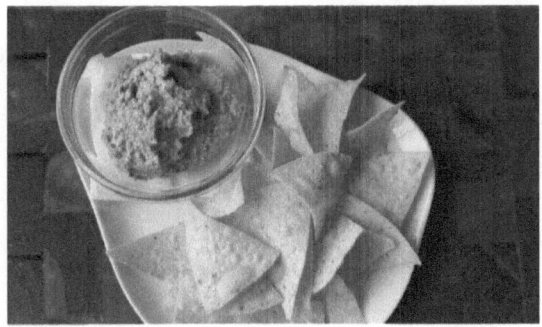

Preparation Time: 11 minutes
Serving size: 4-6

Ingredients

- 12 ounces baby spinach
- 15 oz. cannelloni beans can (rinsed and drained)
- 1 tablespoon lemon juice
- 2 cloves garlic (minced)
- 2 tablespoon olive oil (extra virgin)
- 1 tablespoon vinegar (balsamic)
- ¼ teaspoon black pepper (ground)
- 1 teaspoon salt

Method

1. Heat half the oil in a skillet. Add garlic, cook for a minute. Add half the spinach. Cook for 2 minutes.

2. Add the rest of spinach, and cook till spinach wilts. Leave the mixture to cool.

3. In a food processor, add the spinach mixture, rest of the oil and all the remaining ingredients. Blend till smooth and serve with your choice of bread.

4. BLT with Egg

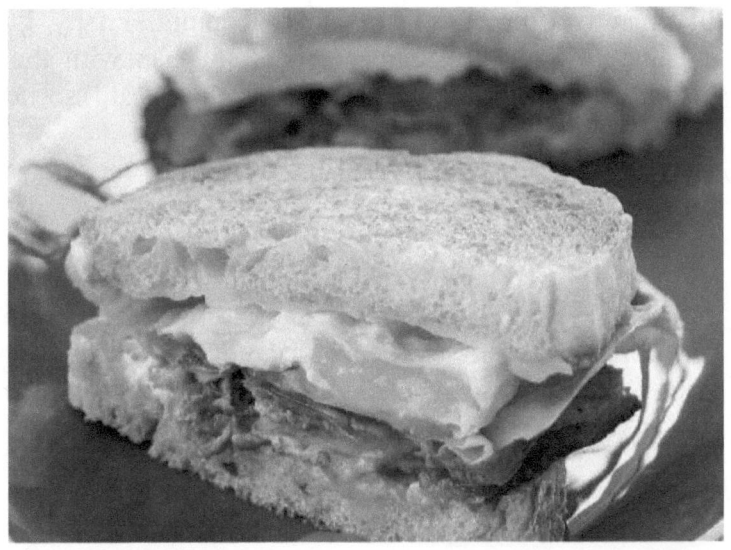

This dish combines the exquisite flavors of a BLT and eggs over easy.

Ingredients

- ☐ 4 slices Bacon
- ☐ 2 large Eggs
- ☐ 4 slices Rye Bread (toasted)
- ● ¼ cup Mayonnaise
- ☐ 2 slices Tomato
- ☐ 1 cup Arugula
- ☐ 1 Tbsp. Chili Sauce
- ☐ Salt & Pepper to taste

Method

1. In a pan over medium heat, cook bacon until crispy. Drain on a paper towel. Cook eggs in the same pan with the bacon drippings. Fry until whites are set but yolk is still soft.

2. Carefully flip the eggs over without cracking the yolk. Cook 1 minute. Remove from heat. Season with salt and pepper to taste.

3. In a bowl, combine mayonnaise and chili sauce. Spread the mayonnaise mixture over each piece of bread. Top each piece with 2 pieces of bacon, a slice of tomato, an egg, and arugula. Cover with the remaining toast. Cut in half.

Health Benefits of Eggs

Despite the rumors, eggs actually lower bad cholesterol. Eggs are packed with muscle-strengthening proteins and B vitamins. Eggs help protect the brain from age-related degeneration.

5. Chicken Empanadas

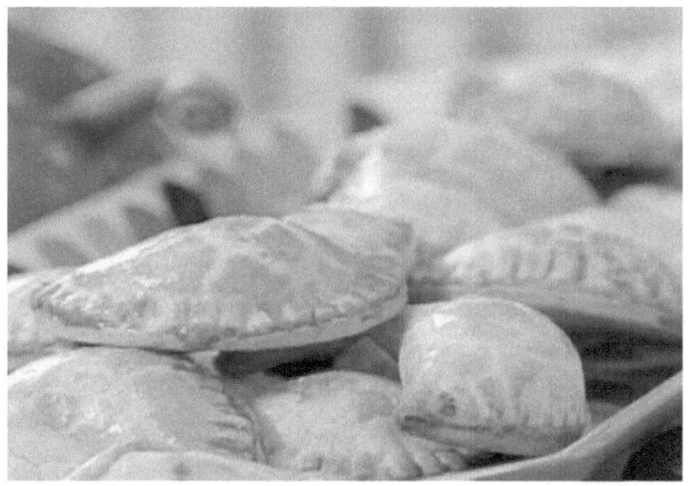

These delicious morsels make a great appetizer or snack.

Ingredients

- 36 Pot-sticker (Gyoza) Wrappers
- ½ lbs. Skinless Boneless Chicken Breasts (cubed)
- ¼ cup Onion (chopped)
- ¼ cup Red Bell Pepper (chopped)
- ¼ cup Tomato (chopped)
- 2 cups Olive Oil
- ¼ cup Water
- 1 clove Garlic (minced)
- 1 large Egg (beaten)

- ☐ 2 Tbsps. Raisins
- ☐ 2 Tbsps. Breadcrumbs
- ☐ 1 Tbsp. Tomato Paste
- ☐ 1 Tbsp. Pimiento-Stuffed Green Olives (chopped)
- ½ tsp Cumin

Method

1. In a large pan on medium-high heat, combine chicken, onion, bell pepper, tomato, garlic, raisins, tomato paste, olives, water, olive oil, and cumin. Cook about 5 minutes.

2. Pour mixture into a food processor and grind coarsely. Mix in breadcrumbs. Refrigerate mixture until cold (about 1 hour). Lay out wrappers on the counter. Lightly brush the edges of the wrappers with egg.

3. Divide mixture evenly among all wrappers. Fold in half. Press edges down with a fork. Heat oil in a large pan on medium-high heat. Add empanadas to hot oil and fry until golden (about 30 seconds each side). Drain on paper towels.

Health Benefits of Olive Oil

Improves circulation. High in unsaturated fats which help you absorb more nutrients, lose weight, and maintain healthy skin. Improves brain health.

Read This FIRST - 100% FREE BONUS

FOR A LIMITED TIME ONLY – Get Olivia's best-selling book *"The #1 Cookbook: Over 170+ of the Most Popular Recipes Across 7 Different Cuisines!"* absolutely FREE!

Readers have absolutely loved this book because of the wide variety of recipes. It is highly recommended you check these recipes out and see what you can add to your home menu!

Once again, as a big thank-you for downloading this book, I'd like to offer it to you *100% FREE for a LIMITED TIME ONLY!*

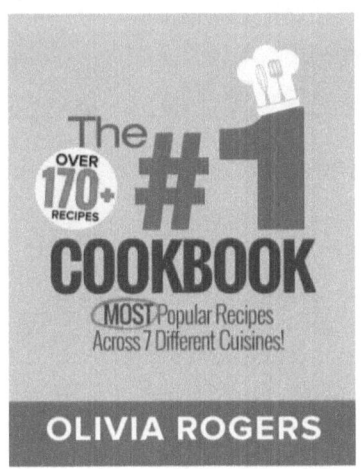

Get your free copy at:

TheMenuAtHome.com/Bonus

6. Open-Faced Radish Sandwiches

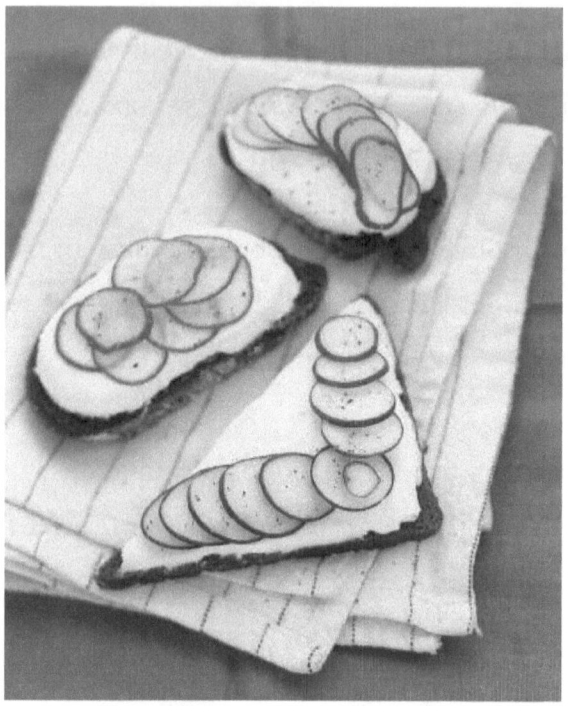

These delightfully simple snacks can be made in under 5 minutes.

Ingredients

- 2 ½ lbs. Radishes
- 20 slices Baguette
- Butter

Method

1. Spread a generous amount of butter on each Baguette slice. Slice radishes thinly. Arrange slices on top of the buttered baguettes.

Health Benefits of Radish

Contains anti-carcinogenic phytochemicals that maintain strong, healthy cells. Helps lower blood pressure. Acts as a natural decongestant.

7. Light Microwave Chips

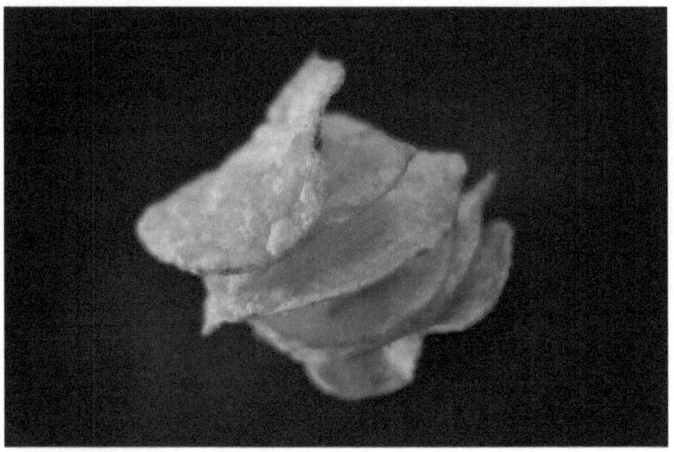

Preparation Time: 45 minutes
Serving size: 4

Ingredients

- 1 1/3 pound of unpeeled, washed potatoes
- ½ teaspoon of salt
- 2 teaspoon olive oil
- Cooking spray

Method

1. Slice the potatoes in to thin slices. Toss salt and oil over the slices evenly. Using a microwave plate, grease it with the cooking spray and lay a layer of potatoes.

2. Microwave for about 3 minutes or until they start turning brown. Turn the slices over, microwave till they are crisp as well as brown around edges.

3. Microwave for about 2-4 more minutes and then lay the chips onto another plate to cool. Repeat with the other slices.

8. Black Bean and Cheese Nachos

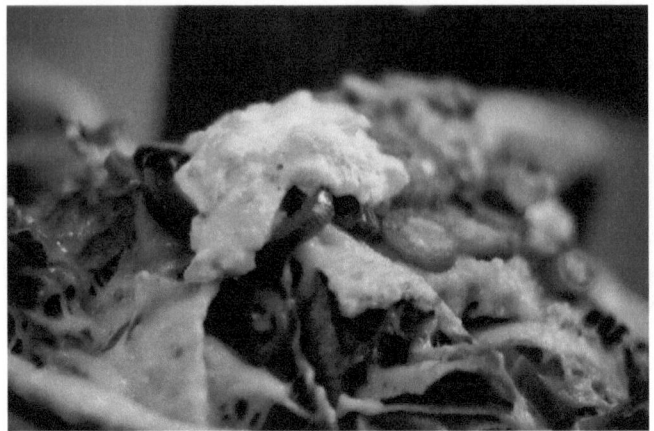

Preparation Time: 30 minutes
Serving size: 4

Ingredients

- ☐ 1 cup Pepper Jack cheese (shredded)
- ☐ 36 low fat baked tortilla chips
- ☐ 14 oz. black beans (rinsed and drained)
- ☐ 2 scallions (sliced thinly)
- ☐ 2 plum tomatoes (chopped)
- • 1 jalapeño pepper (deseeded and diced)
- ☐ 3 tablespoons cilantro (chopped)
- ☐ Lemon wedges
- ☐ Cooking spray

Method

1. Preheat oven at 400F. Use foil to coat baking sheet, grease with cooking spray. Arrange tortilla chips on the baking sheet and sprinkle cheese over them.

2. Now add the tomatoes, beans, scallions and jalapeños over the tortillas and bake for 15-20 minutes till cheese has melted. Remove from oven. Sprinkle and garnish with cilantro. Serve with lemon wedges.

9. Lentil and Carrot Soup

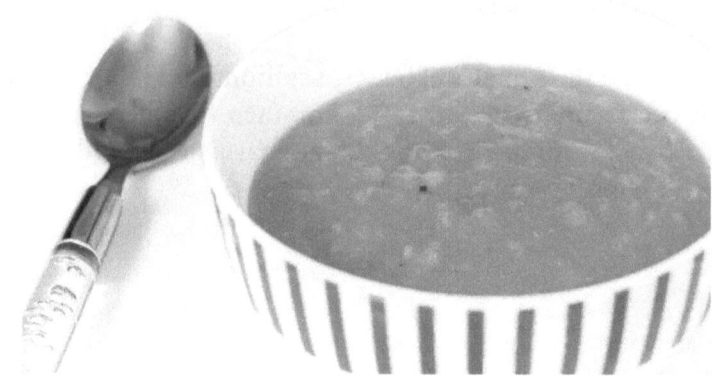

Preparation Time: 25 minutes
Serving size: 2

Ingredients

- 2 teaspoon olive oil
- 1 vegetable stock cube
- 85g red lentils
- 1 onion (sliced)
- 2 carrots (diced)
- 2 tablespoon parsley (chopped)
- 3 sliced garlic cloves
- 1 ¼ liter water

Method

1. Boil water in a kettle. Using a pan, heat oil, fry the onions for 2 minutes. Add garlic and carrots and cook over heat briefly. Pour a liter of boiling water into the pan.

2. Add stock and lentils and stir. Cover pan, cook for 15 minutes till lentils are soft and tender. Take off heat and add parsley. Serve and enjoy!

Section 2: Healthy Meal Options

10. Cauliflower Chicken

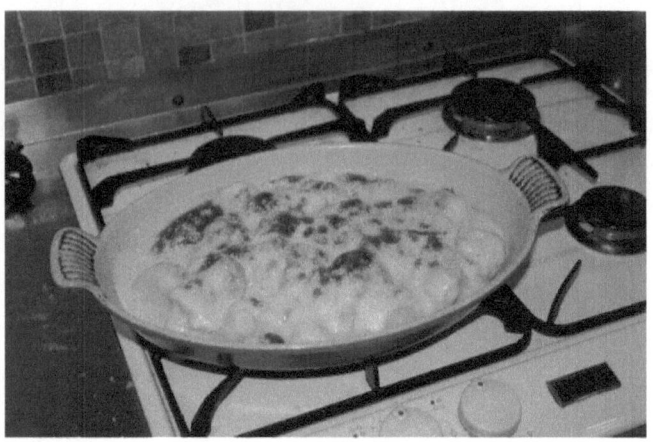

Preparation Time: 35 minutes
Serving size: 3

Ingredients

- ½ pound chicken breast (ground)

- 12 ½ ounce marinara sauce

- 1 head of cauliflower (Chopped)

- ½ onion chopped (fine)

- 2 garlic cloves (minced)

- ½ teaspoon dried oregano

- ½ teaspoon dried parsley

- 1 ½ teaspoon olive oil

- Salt and pepper to taste

- Cooking spray

Method

1. Preheat oven up to 425F degrees. Line baking tray with paper and cover using cooking spray. Toss cauliflower in a bowl, with ¾ teaspoon olive oil, pepper and salt.

2. Place cauliflower in a baking tray and roast for 20 minutes or until golden. Heat oil in a skillet, add garlic and onions, cook for 2 minutes. Then add chicken, parsley, oregano, and cook until chicken is brown stirring with a spoon (wooden).

3. Add marinara sauce to the chicken and let it simmer for about 10-12 minutes. Place each cauliflower in a plate. Top with chicken sauce and serve.

11. Chicken Parmesan

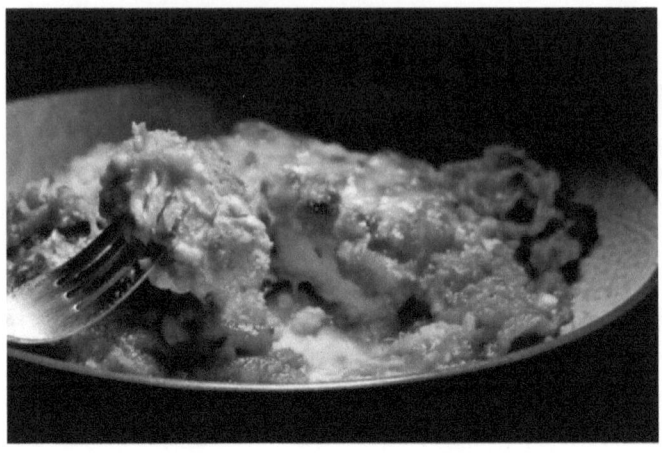

Preparation Time: 50 minutes
Serving size: 2

Ingredients

- 1 zucchini (chopped)//
- ½ pound chicken breast in 4 cutlets (Skinless and Boneless)
- 1 cup broccoli florets
- 1 teaspoon light butter
- ½ teaspoon olive oil
- ¼ teaspoon dried basil
- ¼ cup parmesan cheese (grated)
- 3/8 cup Panko breadcrumbs (Whole Wheat)
- ¼ oregano (dried)

- ¼ parsley (dried)
- ½ teaspoon (garlic powder)
- Pepper and salt to taste
- Cooking Spray

Method

1. Preheat oven up to 375 F degrees. Cover a 9X13 baking dish with spray. Mix parmesan cheese, with breadcrumbs, parsley, garlic powder, oregano, salt, pepper, and basil.

2. Apply butter (melted) on both side of chicken cutlets. For coating, dip the cutlets in the breadcrumbs. Place it in the baking dish.

3. In a bowl, add chopped vegetables while adding olive oil. Add pepper, salt and the breadcrumb mixture. Try to coat evenly. Insert them in the pan with chicken.

4. Bake around 35-40 minutes till chicken is done and cooked throughout. Also check vegetables for tenderness.

12. Sweet & Spicy Shrimp with Noodles

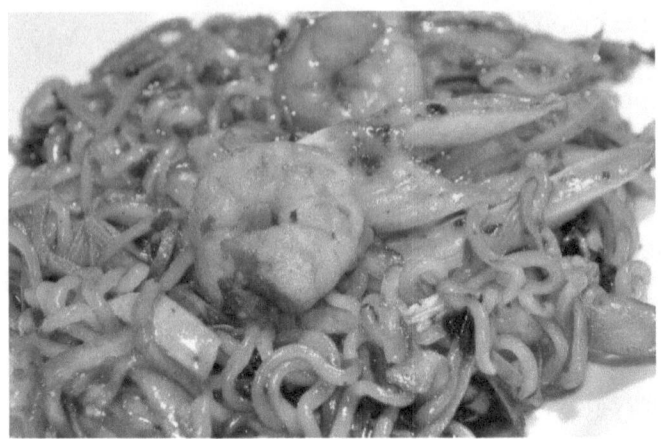

Preparation Time: 60 minutes
Serving size: 2

Ingredients

- ½ tablespoon vinegar (rice)

- ½ tablespoon sambal oelek (like Huy Fong)

- ½ tablespoon low-sodium soy sauce.

- 1 ¼ teaspoon honey

- 6 ounces deveined shrimp (medium size peeled)

- 2-ounce flat rice noodles (uncooked)

- 1 tablespoon unsalted cashews (chopped)

- ½ tablespoon oil (peanut)

- ½ tablespoon sliced garlic (thin)

- 1 teaspoon fresh ginger (peeled and chopped)
- ½ Thai Chile (green, halved)
- 6 mini peppers (sweet, halved)
- 3/8 cup carrot (matchstick cut)
- 1/8 teaspoon salt
- 3/8 cup trimmed snow peas
- 3/8 cup fresh beans (Sprouts)

Method

1. Mix vinegar, honey, sambal oelek and soy sauce in a medium bowl while stirring with a whisk. Add shrimp to the mixture, and coat them. Refrigerate them while covered for 30 minutes.

2. Prepare noodles as per packet direction. Leave fat and salt for now. Wash in cold water, then drain. Heat a skillet (large) on medium to high heat. Insert oil in pan, and mix to coat. Add garlic, chile, cashew and ginger in pan. Fry while stirring for 1 minute or till brown.

3. Remove the mixture from pan and keep it aside. Raise the heat temperature. Now add carrot, sweet peppers, and salt in pan. Fry and stir for 2 minutes. Add the mixture (shrimp) in it. (Don't drain).

4. Fry and stir for another 2 minutes. Add peas and noodles in it. Cook 1 minute. Toss and mix to coat. Add cashew mixture and bean sprouts in the pan and cook for 1 minute. Toss frequently and serve.

13. Grilled Chicken with Salad and Pineapple Dressing

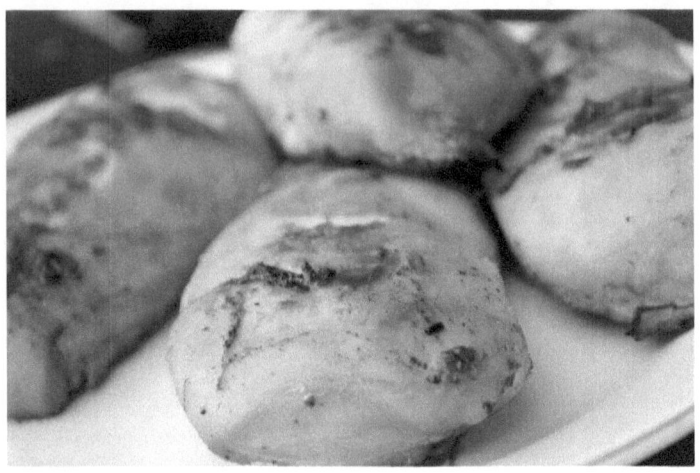

Preparation Time: 20 minutes
Serving size: 2

Ingredients

- ½ pound chicken breast (skinless)
- 4-ounce fresh pineapple (cut into 1-inch cubes)
- 4 cups baby spinach
- 1 tablespoon cilantro (chopped)
- 3/8 jicama (peeled, julienne)
- ¼ cup onion (sliced)
- 1/3 cup red bell pepper (sliced)
- ½ clove of garlic

- ¼ teaspoon habanero pepper (minced)
- ½ teaspoon chili powder
- ¼ teaspoon salt
- 1 tablespoon orange juice
- 2 teaspoon apple cider vinegar
- 1/8 cup olive oil
- Cooking spray
- Plastic wrap

Method

1. Wrap chicken in plastic wrap and flatten to even thickness. Remove wrap. Sprinkle chicken with chili powder and salt. Coat with cooking spray.

2. Heat a pan and place chicken on it. Cook each side for 3 minutes. Remove from pan. Blend half of cilantro, pineapple, vinegar, juice, habanero and garlic, till smooth. Gradually add olive oil until blend well.

3. Mix all remaining ingredients in a bowl and add ¾ of the blended dressing and toss. Divide salad onto plates, add thinly cut slices of chicken and drizzle remaining dressing. Serve.

14. Citrus Beef Kebabs

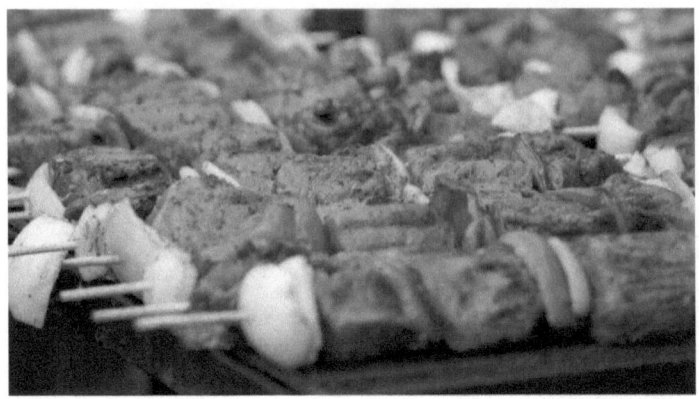

Preparation Time: 40 minutes
Serving size: 2

Ingredients

- ½ pound sirloin steak boneless (1-inch pieces)
- ½ orange
- 2 cups watermelon, plums, peaches and/or mango (cubed)
- 1/8 cup cilantro (chopped)
- ½ tablespoon paprika (smoked)
- 1/8 teaspoon red pepper (ground)
- Salt to taste
- Bamboo skewers (4)
- Coal grill

Method

1. Extract 1 tablespoon from orange and keep aside. Mix orange peel, paprika, cilantro and red pepper. Mix beef and half of the above mixture in a zip lock bag.

2. Place remaining mixture and fruits into a separate bag and mix. Keep fruit and beef in the fridge for 15-30 minutes. Thread beef into 2 skewers, leaving some space in between.

3. Thread fruit into 2 skewers. Place kabobs on to coals and grill. Beef for 8-10 minutes and fruit till they soften or brown. Season with salt and drizzle over orange juice. Serve.

15. Thai Prawns with Pineapple Rice

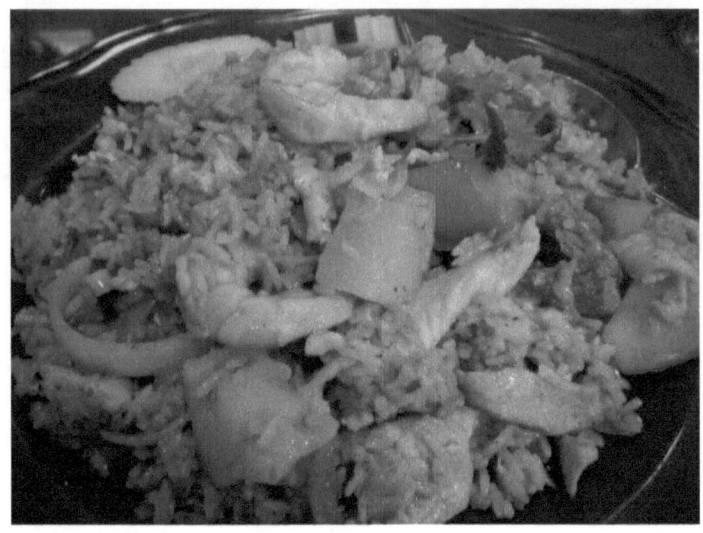

Preparation Time: 25 minutes
Serving size: 2

Ingredients

- 1 teaspoon sunflower oil
- Spring onions, white and green separated (sliced)
- ½ green pepper (Chopped and deseeded)
- 70 grams pineapple (Chopped)
- 1 ½ tablespoon Thai curry (green paste)
- 2 teaspoon soy sauce (light)
- 150 grams, basmati rice (cooked) OR 70-gram uncooked rice
- 1 egg (large and beaten)

- 70-gram frozen peas

- 113 grams, drained bamboo shoots (can)

- 125 g frozen pawns (raw or cooked)

- 1 – 1 ½ limes, (½ juiced, 1 wedged)

- Coriander leaves (handful)

Method

1. Heat oil in a pan. Add whites of green onion. Fry for 2 minutes. Add pepper, and after 1 min add pineapple. Add green paste and soy sauce after 1 minute. Add rice and stir-fry and separate on a side of pan.

2. Scramble eggs on the other side. Stir in the peas, prawns and bamboo. Heat for 2 minutes till peas are tender. Add spring onions green, lime juice, and coriander. Serve with lime wedges and soy sauce.

16. Asparagus and Potato Frittatas

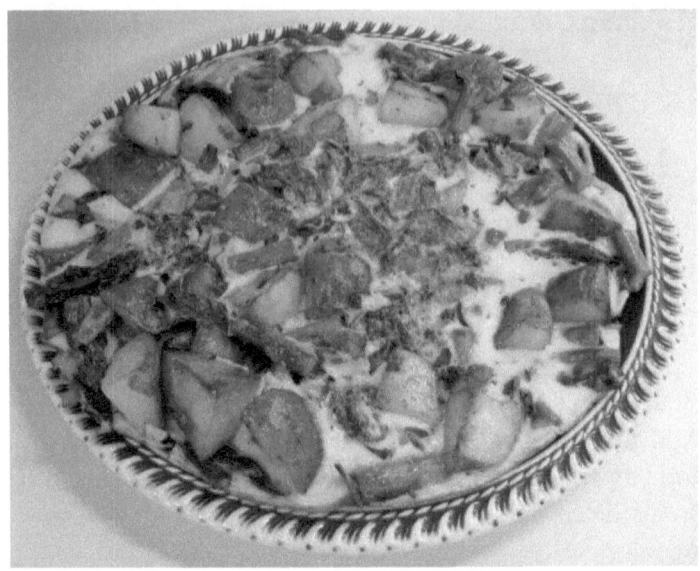

Preparation Time: 22 minutes
Serving size: 3

Ingredients

- ☐ 6 eggs beaten

- ☐ 200-gram potatoes (quartered)

- ☐ 40-gram grated cheddar

- ☐ 100-gram asparagus

- ☐ Rocket leaves

- ☐ 1 onion (chopped fine)

- ☐ Cold salted water

Method

1. Boil potatoes in cold salted water until tender. Add asparagus for a minute and then drain. Heat oil and add onion. Cook till soft approximately 8 minutes. Mix eggs and half the cheese.

2. Pour egg mixture over onions and then scatter over potatoes. Top with remaining cheese and put pan on grill for 5 minutes or till golden brown. Cut into wedges and serve.

17. Fish Stew

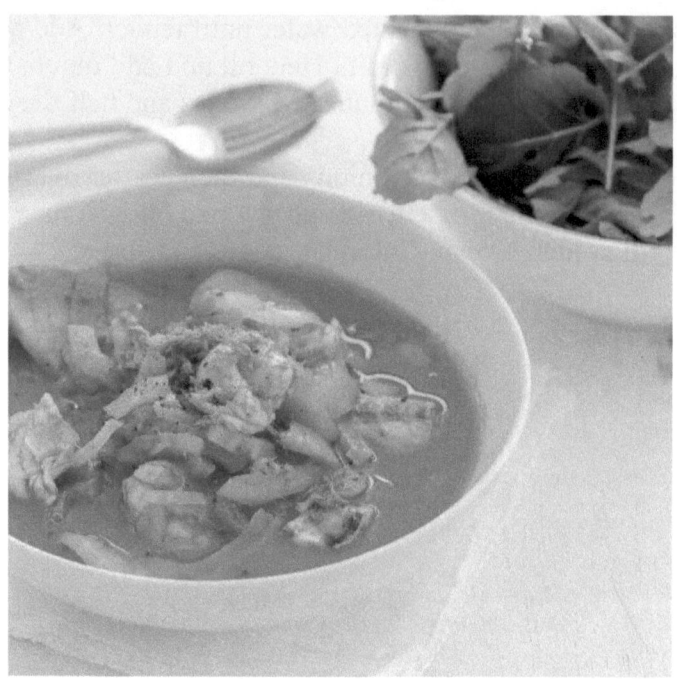

Preparation Time: 35 minutes
Serving size: 2

Ingredients

- ☐ 85 grams shelled king prawns
- ☐ 200 grams Pollock fillets (skinless and cut in chunks)
- ☐ 500 ml fish stock
- ☐ 2 carrots (diced)
- ☐ 2 garlic cloves (chopped)
- ☐ 400-gram tomatoes (chopped)

- 2 leeks (sliced)
- 2 diced celery sticks
- 1 teaspoon fennel seeds
- 1 tablespoon olive oil
- Salt and pepper (seasoning)

Method

1. Heat oil in a pan and add carrot, celery, garlic and fennel seeds. Cook till they start to soften and then add leek, tomatoes and stock and season.

2. Let it boil then cover and simmer for 15-20 minutes till veggies are tender and sauce thickens. Add fish and prawns. Cook for 2 more minutes and serve.

18. Red Pepper Chicken

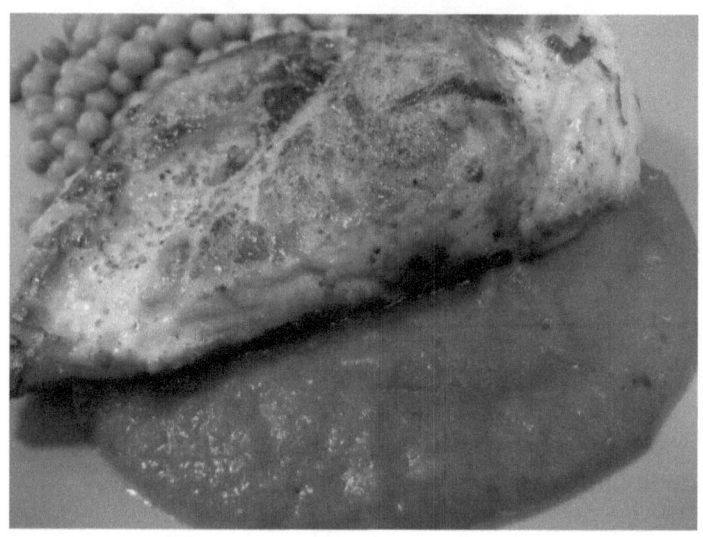

Preparation Time: 35 minutes
Serving size: 2

Ingredients

- ½ tablespoon light butter
- 1/8 cup onion (chopped)
- 1 clove garlic (minced)
- 7 ½ ounce roasted red peppers (canned, drained, chopped)
- ¼ teaspoon red pepper (crushed)
- 1/8 cup basil leaves (chopped)
- ½ pound chicken breast
- 2-ounce fat-free cream cheese

- Salt and pepper to taste

Method

1. Melt butter in pan and add chicken. Cook for 5 minutes and then remove chicken and keep aside. Sauté garlic and onion with butter for 2-3 minutes.

2. Add peppers and sauté for 2 minutes. Add cream cheese, crushed peppers and broth and let it simmer for 10-15 minutes till cream cheese melts and sauce thickens.

3. Stir in basil, and cook for 2 more minutes. Season with salt and pepper. Pour red pepper sauce over chicken and serve.

19. Moroccan Veggie Stew

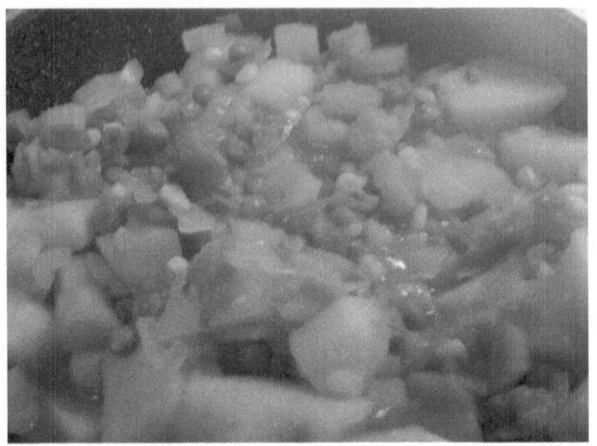

Preparation Time: 65 minutes
Serving size: 2

Ingredients

- ½ onion (finely sliced)
- 1 leek (trimmed and sliced)
- 1 garlic clove (finely sliced)
- 200g tomatoes (chopped)
- ½ yellow pepper (deseeded and cut in chunks)
- ½ red pepper (deseeded and cut into chunks)
- 185g sweet potatoes in chunks (peeled)
- ¼ pack coriander (chopped)
- ½ orange juice and peel

- 200g chickpeas (drained and rinsed)
- 50-gram lentils (dried and split)
- 25 g mixed nuts roughly chopped and toasted (pecans, hazelnuts, walnuts, brazil nut)
- 1 teaspoon coriander (ground)
- 1 teaspoon cumin (ground)
- ¼ teaspoon chili flakes
- A pinch of cinnamon (ground)
- ½ tablespoon rapeseed oil
- Ground black pepper
- 200ml water
- Yogurt to serve

Method

1. Heat oil in saucepan, and gently fry leeks and onion for 10-15 minutes until soft. Add garlic and cook for 2 more minutes.
2. Stir in cumin, cinnamon, chili and coriander. And cook for 2 minutes, stir frequently. Season with black pepper.
3. Add peppers, lentils, chickpeas, tomatoes, orange juice and peel, sweet potatoes and half the nuts.
4. Add water, let it simmer and cook for 15 minutes, till potatoes soften but not breaking. Serve, and garnish with nuts, yogurt and coriander.

20. Meatloaf

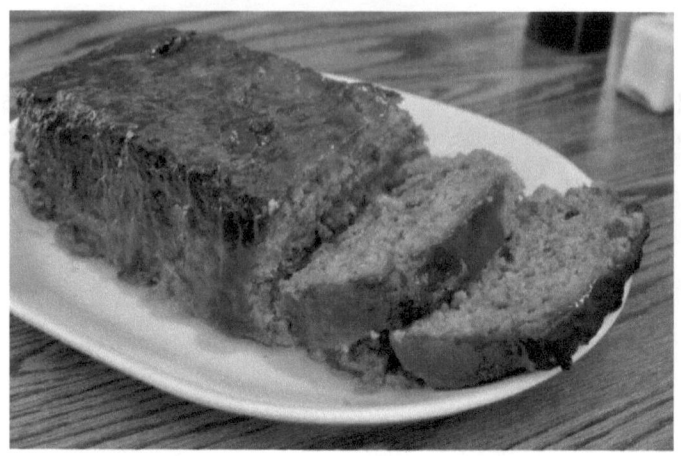

Preparation Time: 10 minutes (ready in 70 minutes)
Serving size: 8

Ingredients

- 1 ½ pound lean beef (ground
- 1 egg
- 1 cup low fat (1%) milk
- 1 cup bread crumbs (whole wheat)
- 1 onion (chopped)
- ½ cup parsley (chopped)
- 1 carrot (grated)
- 1 tablespoon sugar (brown)
- 2 tablespoon mustard

- 1/3 cup ketchup

- Salt and pepper (to taste)

Method

1. Preheat oven to 350F degrees. Lightly grease 9x5 loaf pan. Mix beef, onion, egg, milk, bread crumbs, carrot and parsley. Season with salt and pepper.

2. Put mixture in pan. Stir sugar, ketchup and mustard together and pour over meat loaf. Bake in oven for about an hour (thermometer inserted in center should read 160F degrees).

Section 3: Sweet on The Tooth, Light on The Tummy

21. Cheesecake Brownies

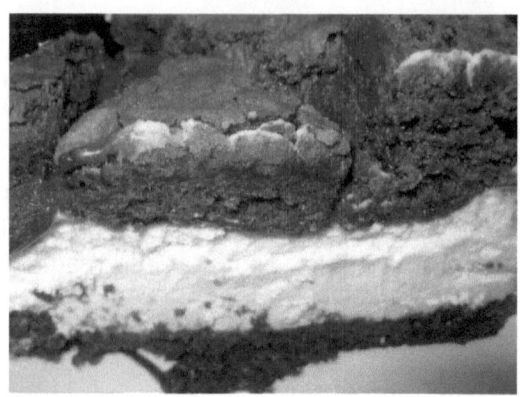

Preparation Time: 2 hrs 30 minutes (active time 25 minutes)
Serving size: 24

Ingredients

- ¼ cup normal sugar
- 4 ounces cream cheese (low fat)
- 2 eggs (large)
- 1 tablespoon flour (all-purpose)
- ½ teaspoon extract (vanilla)
- 1 tablespoon yogurt (non-fat, plain)
- 2/3 cup pastry flour (whole-wheat)
- ½ cup cocoa powder (unsweetened)

- 2 egg whites
- ¼ teaspoon natural salt
- 1 ¼ cup sugar (light brown and packed)
- ¼ cup oil (canola)
- 2 teaspoon extract (vanilla)
- ¼ cup coffee/black tea (strong or instant)
- Spray (cooking)

Method

1. Preheat your oven to 350F degrees. Spray a 7 x 11-inch baking pan.

2. Topping: Using an electric beater, beat cream cheese till its creamy and smooth. Then add the sugar and beat into smoothness. Add flour, egg, vanilla and yogurt and beat till it is blended smoothly.

3. Brownie layer: Using a bowl, whisk the flour salt and cocoa. In another bowl beat the egg, brown sugar and egg whites till its smooth. Add coffee, oil and vanilla, and then add the other dry ingredients. Keep beating till well blended, scraping the sides.

4. Put half the brownie batter in the baking pan. Then pour the cream topping over the brownie. Add large dollops of the left-over brownie batter. Create a swirl effect with a skewer or knife. Bake for approximately 20 minutes, till the brownies are firm. Cool and serve!

22. Power Bars

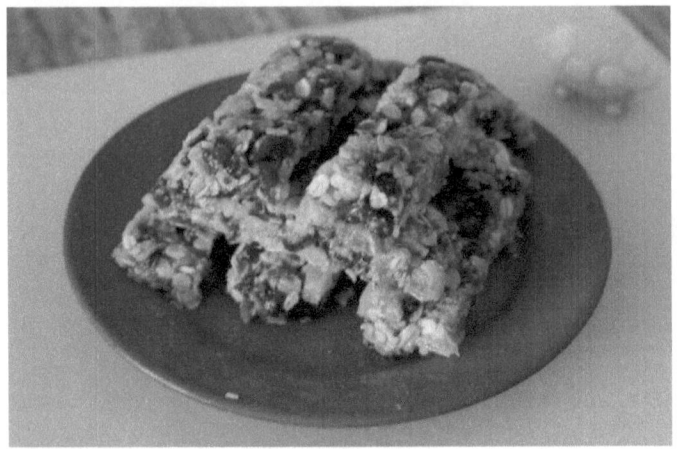

Preparation Time: 20 minutes
Serving size: 12

Ingredients

- 1/2 tablespoon flaxseeds (golden)
- ½ tablespoon of sesame seeds
- 1/3 cup of sunflower seeds
- 1/6 teaspoon of salt
- ¼ teaspoon extract (vanilla)
- ¼ cup honey
- ¼ cup of almond butter
- 1/3 cup currants
- 1/ cup peanuts (dry roasted variety)

- 1/3 cup apricots (dried and chopped)

- 1 cup of rolled oats

- 1cup puffed cereal (unsweetened, whole grain)

Method

1. Preheat oven to 350F degrees. In a bowl, mix peanuts, all 3 seeds and oats. Transfer on to a greased baking dish. Bake the oat mixture till the oats start to toast. Shake pan for approximately 10 minutes. Transfer back into the bowl.

2. Add cereal, apricots, raisins and currants and mix slightly. Using a saucepan, mix the butter, salt, honey and extract. Keep stirring frequently till the mixture bubbles.

3. Add sauce to the oat and raisin mixture and mix. Transfer onto a greased pan. Pressing the mixture into a layer, then put it into the fridge to cool and become firm. Cut into slices and serve!

23. Chia Seed Yogurt

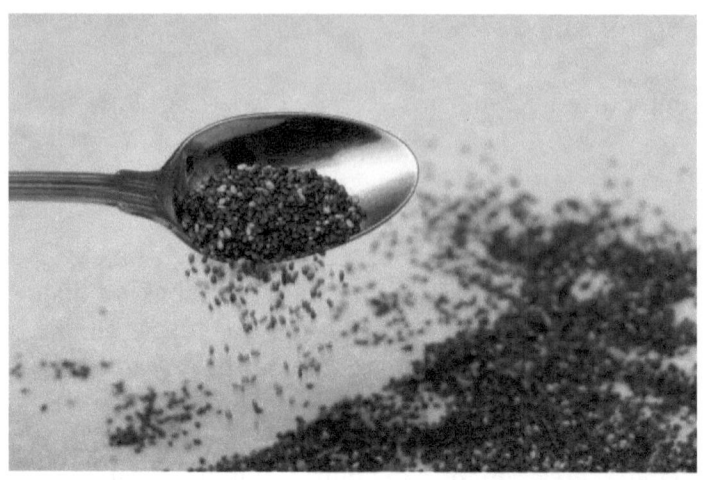

Preparation Time: 4 hours (5 minutes active time)
Serving size: 2

Ingredients

- ☐ 1 cup Greek Yogurt (nonfat, plain)
- ☐ 1 cup milk (nonfat)
- ¼ cup of chia seeds
- ¼ teaspoon vanilla extract
- ¼ teaspoon of cinnamon (ground)
- ☐ Sweetener of your liking

Method

1. Stir all the ingredients together in a bowl. Cover the bowl and keep it in the refrigerator for about 4 hours. Enjoy!

24. Blueberry Cobbler

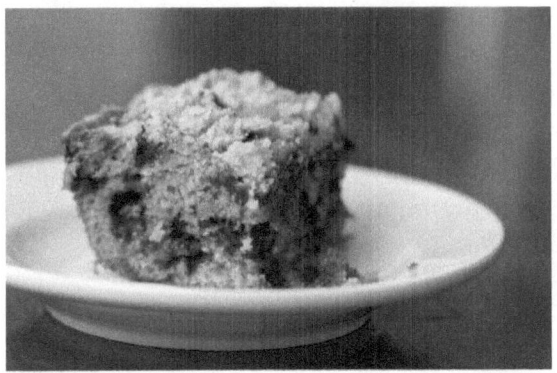

Preparation Time: 30 minutes
Serving size: 2

Ingredients

- 1 ½ cup blueberries
- I teaspoon lemon juice
- 1 teaspoon lemon zest (grated)
- ¼ teaspoon cinnamon
- 2 tablespoons sugar
- 1 teaspoon crystallized ginger (minced)
- ½ cup bisquick (baking mix)
- ½ teaspoon icing sugar
- 3 tablespoons skimmed milk
- Nonstick spray

Method

1. Preheat your oven to 450F degrees. Spray 2 custard cups (6 ounce). Mix sugar, blueberries, lemon zest, ginger, cinnamon and lemon juice.

2. Pour half into each cup. Mix milk and bisquick in a bowl. Ladle over the blueberry mixture. Sprinkle with icing sugar. Bake for 20 minutes or till golden. Enjoy!

25. Chocolate and Zucchini Bread

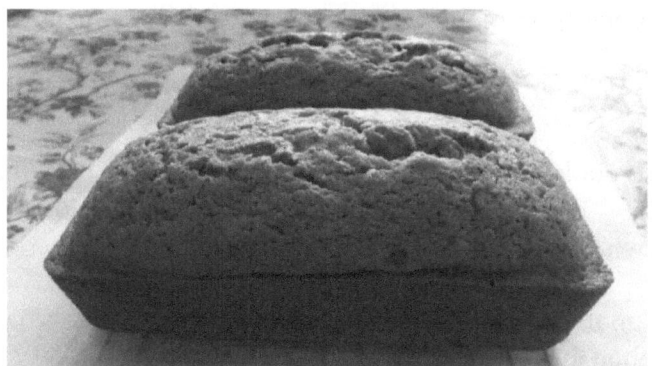

Preparation Time: 50-60 minutes
Serving size: 16

Ingredients

- Spray (Cooking)

- 1 cup flour (unbleached whole wheat)

- ½ cup sugar (brown – not packed)

- ½ teaspoon salt

- 1 1/8 teaspoon baking soda

- ½ cup chocolate chips

- 1 teaspoon vanilla

- 1 beaten large egg

- 1 cup sauce (apple)

- 1 teaspoon vanilla

- 1 ½ cup zucchini (shredded – not packed)
- 2 tablespoon melted butter

Method

1. Use cooking spray on 9" x 5" loaf pan. Pre-heat the oven to 325 F degrees. Mix sugar, salt, flour and baking soda in a bowl. Insert Chocolate chips to the batter.

2. In another bowl, add vanilla, apple sauce, egg, zucchini and melted better. Mix and stir it with the batter. Now add the batter into loaf pan.

3. Now bake it for 40-50 minutes and keep checking the center of the cake with a toothpick for its consistency. Let it sit for 10 minutes to cool. Remove from the pan and the serving is ready.

Section 4: Energizing Healthy Beverages

26. Pumpkin Smoothie

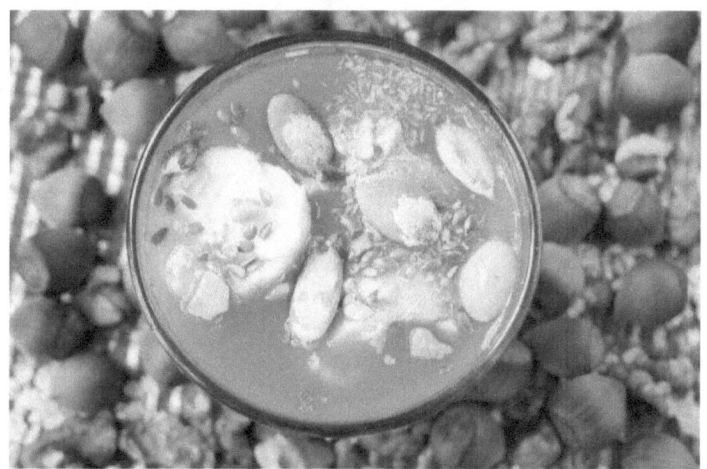

Preparation Time: 5 minutes
Serving size: 2

Ingredients

- 1 banana
- 1 cup unsweetened almond vanilla
- 1 teaspoon pumpkin pie spice
- ½ cup greek yogurt (nonfat, vanilla flavored)
- ½ cup canned pumpkin
- 1 tablespoon vanilla extract
- Ice cubes (4-5)

Method

1. Take a blender and pour all ingredients. Blend till smooth. Serve and enjoy!

27. Green Concoction

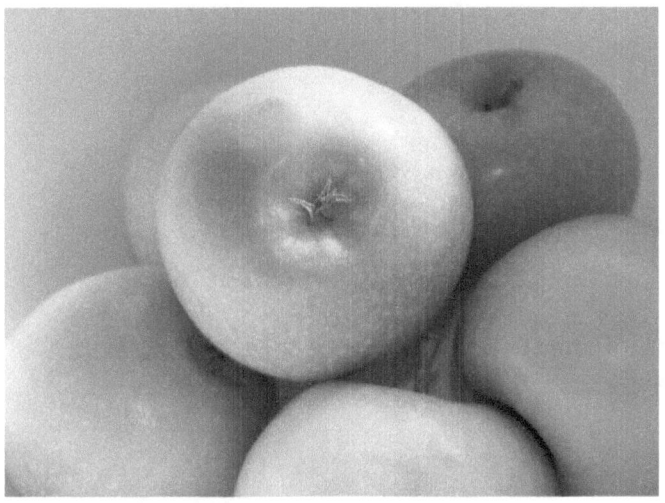

Preparation Time: 10 minutes
Serving size: 2

Ingredients

- 2 green apples (cut in halves)
- 4 celery stalks
- 1 cucumber
- 6 kale leaves
- ½ lemon (peeled)
- 1-inch fresh ginger

Method

1. Process all the above ingredients in a juicer and enjoy!

28. Citrus Coconut Water

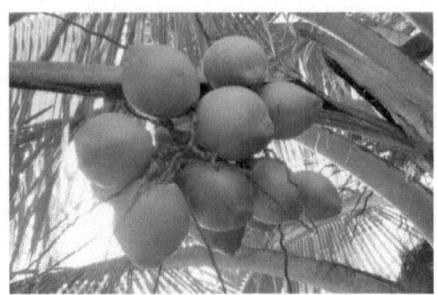

Preparation Time: 10 minutes
Serving size: 2

Ingredients

- 2 tablespoons freshly squeezed lime juice
- 2 cups water (coconut)
- ½ cup freshly squeezed orange juice
- 2 teaspoon sugar
- ¼ cup freshly squeezed lemon juice
- Some ice (1 cup)
- Orange slices, lemon or lime

Method

1. Add the ingredients in a blender (do not add sliced fruits at this stage). Blend till everything is incorporated.

2. Pour in the container and use the sliced fruits as topping. Drink is ready to be served with citrus slices.

29. Frappuccino

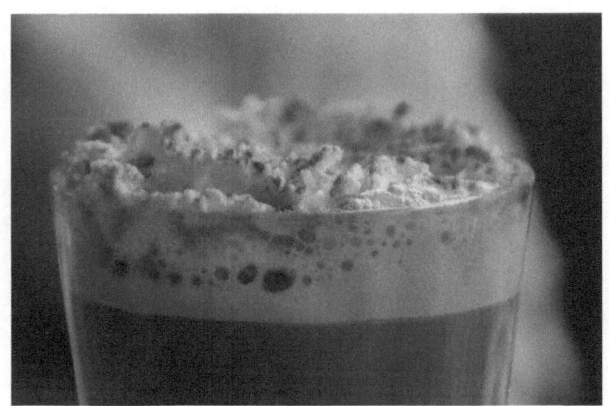

Preparation Time: 2 minutes
Serving size: 1

Ingredients

- ½ cup milk (fat free)
- 2 tablespoon coffee granules (decaf or regular)
- Some Ice-cubes (7-9)
- 2 tablespoon vanilla creamer for coffee (powdered, fat free)
- Sweetener/toppings (if desired)

Method

1. Add these ingredients in a mixture/blender. Incorporate till it gets smooth.
2. Use sweetener or toppings according to the taste. Pour in the container and serve.

30. Wasabi Tuna Kebabs

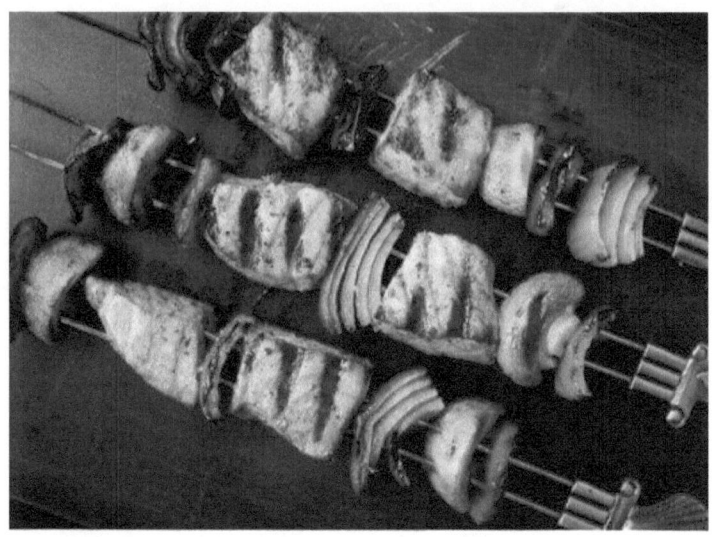

These kebabs combine the subtlety of tuna with the boldness of wasabi and pepper to create a perfectly balanced dish.

Ingredients

- ☐ 28 Wooden Skewers
- ☐ 1 lbs. Tuna Steaks (cubed)
- ½ cup Mayonnaise
- ☐ 28 slices Pickled Ginger
- ☐ 1 bunch Watercress
- 2 ½ Tbsps. Soy Sauce
- ☐ 2 Tbsps. Wasabi Powder
- ☐ 1 Tbsp. Olive Oil

- 1 ½ tsp Water

- 1 tsp Pepper

Method

1. In a bowl, blend wasabi powder and water. Whisk in mayonnaise. Refrigerate 30 minutes. In another bowl, combine tuna and soy sauce. Toss to coat. Let marinate 30 minutes at room temperature. Stir occasionally.

2. Slide 1 ginger slice onto each skewer (about 2" from the tip). Line a platter with watercress. Place the wasabi mayonnaise bowl on the platter. Drain tuna. Pat dry. Return to bowl. Sprinkle tuna with pepper. Toss to coat.

3. In a large pan over medium-high heat, heat oil. Sear tuna (browned on the outside, pink inside). Remove from heat. Slide a piece of tuna onto each skewer next to the ginger. Arrange skewers on platter.

Health Benefits of Wasabi

Acts as a natural remedy for infection and inflammation. Inhibits the growth of cavity-causing bacteria in the mouth. Helps the body break down and eliminate toxins.

31. Puff Pastry Pizza

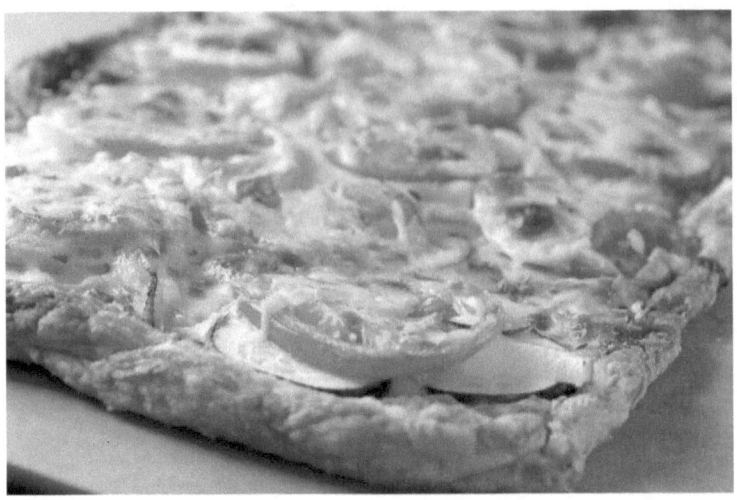

Puff pastry, tuna, and fresh basil transform this surprisingly simple dish into a delicacy.

Ingredients

- ☐ 1 sheet Puff Pastry
- ½ lbs. Tuna Steak (sliced)
- ☐ 4 large Green Onions (chopped)
- ☐ 4 oz. Mozzarella (thinly sliced)
- ☐ 12 large Fresh Basil Leaves
- ☐ 4 Cherry Tomatoes (quartered)
- ☐ 4 Olives (pitted, quartered)
- ☐ 2 Radishes (sliced)

- 2 tsp Olive Oil

- 1 tsp Fresh Ginger (peeled, minced)

Method

1. Preheat oven to 400°F. On a floured surface, roll out puff pastry to an 11" square. Cut out 4 ½" rounds from the pastry. Transfer to ungreased baking sheet. Place another baking sheet on top to weigh down the pastry rounds. Bake until golden brown (about 20 minutes). Uncover and let cool completely. Leave oven on.

2. Heat 2 teaspoons olive oil in a pan on medium heat. Add green onions. Cook 2 minutes. Remove from heat. Sprinkle green onions on pastry rounds. Light brush tuna with olive oil. Sprinkle with salt and pepper to taste.

3. Place 3 slices tuna, 3 slices mozzarella, and 3 basil leaves on each pastry (alternate the slices so that you have a tuna-mozzarella-basil pattern). Sprinkle the tops with ginger and olive oil. Bake about 3 minutes.

Health Benefits of Tuna

High in Omega-3s which protect your heart and brain. Helps lower blood pressure and stabilize blood sugar. Stimulates the metabolism and speeds up weight loss.

32. Garlic Chili Shrimp

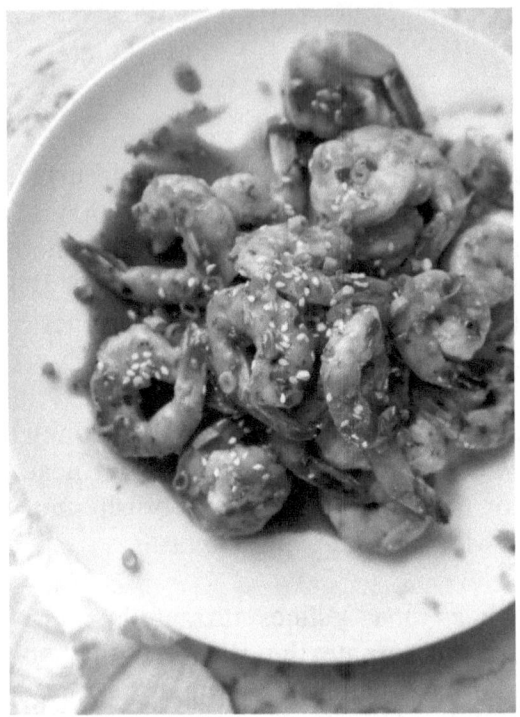

Whip up this delicious shrimp lunch or dinner in under 15 minutes.

Ingredients

- ☐ 1 lbs. Small Shrimp (peeled, deveined)
- ½ cup Olive Oil
- ☐ 4 cloves Garlic (chopped)
- ☐ 1 tsp Crushed Red Pepper Flakes
- ☐ Salt to taste
- ☐ Crusty Bread

Method

1. Heat ¼ cup oil in a large pan on medium heat. Add 2 garlic cloves and ½ teaspoon crushed red pepper flakes. Cook 1 minute.

2. Lightly salt ½ lbs. shrimp. Add to pan. Cook 1-2 minutes. Transfer shrimp with oil to a bowl. Repeat with the remaining oil, garlic, red pepper flakes, and shrimp. Return first batch of shrimp and oil to pan. Toss to mix. Serve with crusty bread.

Health Benefits of Garlic

Eat raw garlic to treat infections (bacterial and viral). Remove warts by apply raw garlic directly onto the wart (do this for 15 minutes twice daily). Eat garlic before your workouts to reduce muscle fatigue and improve your endurance.

33. Tuna & White Bean Salad

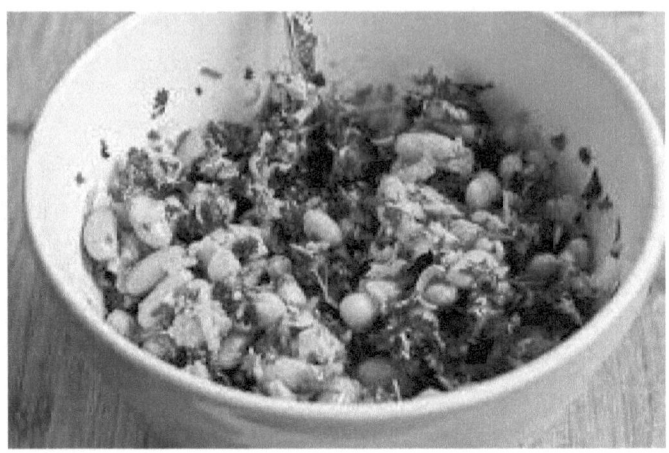

This quick layered salad is a fantastic lunch or side dish for your dinner.

Ingredients

- ☐ 1 cup Canned Tuna (drain, broken into pieces)
- ☐ 2 (15oz.) cans White Beans (drained, rinsed)
- ☐ 1 head Radicchio (cored, leaves chopped)
- ☐ 2 stalks Celery (thinly sliced)
- ☐ 6 Tbsps. Parsley Vinaigrette
- ☐ Salt & Pepper to taste

Method

1. In a large bowl, combine radicchio and 3 tablespoons vinaigrette. Toss to coat. Season with salt and pepper to taste. Arrange on a serving platter.

2. In the bowl, combine 3 tablespoons vinaigrette with beans and celery. Toss to coat. Season with salt and pepper to taste. Arrange mixture on top of radicchios. Top with tuna. Drizzle a little more vinaigrette over everything.

Health Benefits of White Beans

High in the detoxifying mineral "molybdenum." Prevent body from storing excess body fat. High in muscle-building magnesium.

34. Summery Shrimp Salad

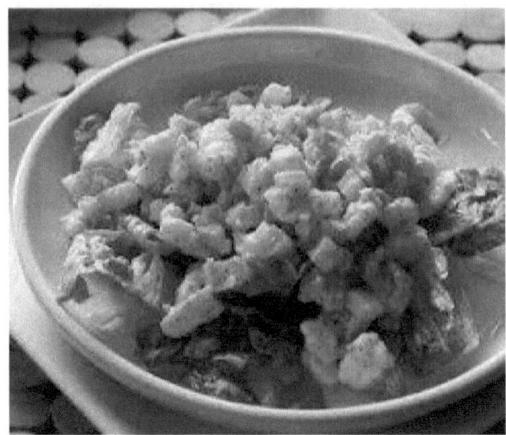

Enjoy the richly complex range of flavors in this dish which can be prepared in under 30 minutes.

Ingredients

- ☐ 4 cups Rice (cooked)
- ☐ 1 lbs. Medium Shrimp (peeled, deveined)
- ☐ 2 Zucchini (halved, sliced)
- ½ Lemon (thinly sliced)
- ½ Lemon (juiced)
- ☐ 1 cup Wax Beans
- ☐ 1 cup Green Beans
- ☐ 1 cup Snap Peas (halved)
- ½ cup Peas

- 3 Tbsps. Olive Oil
- 1 bulb Fennel (thinly sliced)
- 1 tsp Paprika
- 1 tsp Chili Powder
- 1 tsp Cayenne Pepper
- ½ tsp Garlic Powder
- ½ tsp Coriander
- ½ tsp Cumin

Method

1. In a bowl, mix olive oil with cayenne, paprika, chili powder, coriander, garlic powder, and cumin. Add shrimp. Toss to coat. Heat ½ tablespoon oil in a pan on medium heat. Add lemon slices. Cook until golden. Remove and set aside.

2. Increase heat to high and add remaining oil to pan. Add shrimp. Cook 1 minute. Add fennel, green beans, wax beans, peas, and snap peas. Cook 1 minute. Stir in lemon slices and lemon juice. Serve over rice.

Health Benefits of Shrimp

Just 6oz. of shrimp contains 39 grams of protein. It also contains 35% of your zinc and more than 100% of your selenium. B vitamins in shrimp help maintain healthy red blood cells.

35. Crispy Artichokes in Aged Balsamic

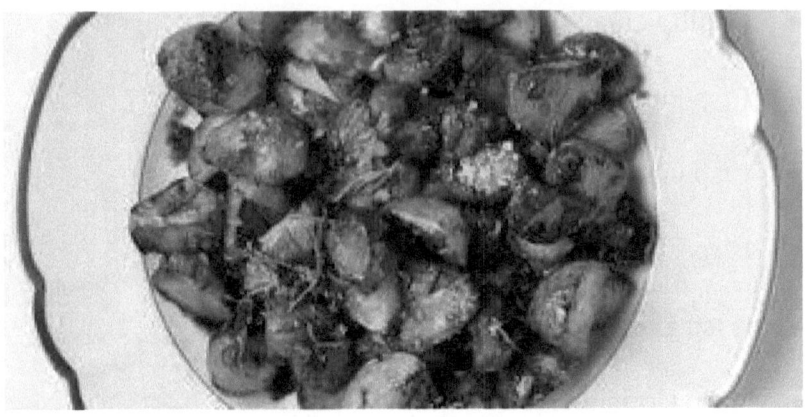

This is an absolutely exquisite side dish or appetizer that can be thrown together in under 30 minutes!

Ingredients

- ☐ 2 lbs. Artichokes (scrubbed, quartered)
- ¼ cup Butter
- ¼ cup Water
- ☐ 3 Tbsps. Aged Balsamic Vinegar
- ☐ 2 Tbsps. Olive Oil
- ☐ 4 sprigs Rosemary
- ☐ Salt & Pepper to taste

Method

1. Heat oil in a large pan over medium-high heat. Add artichokes and water. Season with salt and pepper to taste. Cover and cook 8-10 minutes, stirring occasionally. Uncover and

continue cooking until water is evaporated and artichokes are crisp. Transfer to a platter.

2. In the pan, combine butter and rosemary. Cook until butter browns (about 4 minutes). Remove from heat. Mix in vinegar. Spoon the butter mixture over the artichokes.

Health Benefits of Artichoke

High in folate. High in fiber. High in antioxidants (ranked #7 on the list of foods highest in antioxidants).

36. Winter Squash Soup with Pumpkin Seeds

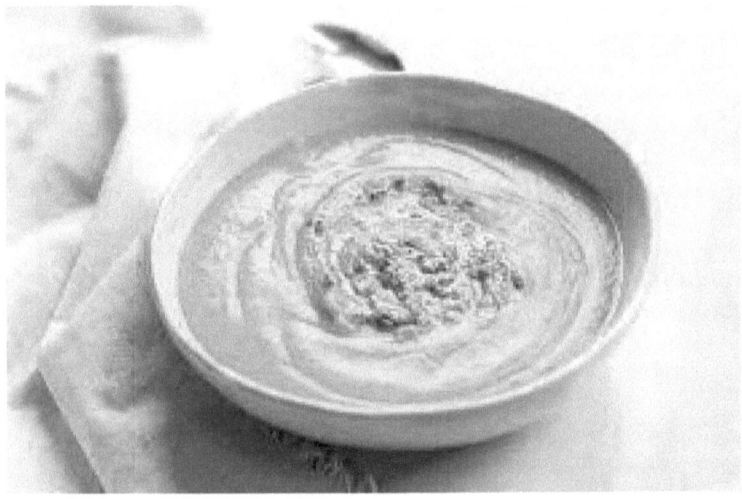

This rich soup warms you to the bones and leaves you satisfied for hours.

Ingredients

- 3 cups Chicken Stock
- 2 (12oz.) packages Frozen Winter Squash Puree
- 3 Shallots (chopped)
- 1 Tbsp. Butter
- ¾ cup Raw Pumpkin Seeds
- 1 Tbsp. Olive Oil
- 1 tsp Cayenne Pepper
- ¾ tsp Cumin

- 1 tsp Lime Zest

- 1 Tbsp. Fresh Lime Juice

Method

1. Melt butter in a large pot on medium-high heat. Add shallots. Cook 3 minutes. Stir in stock and squash puree. Reduce heat and simmer 30 minutes (uncovered).

2. While simmering, heat oil in a small pan on medium-high heat. Add pumpkin seeds. Cook 1-2 minutes, stirring constantly. Seeds will begin to pop. Stir in cayenne pepper and cumin. Continue stirring about 30 seconds.

3. Transfer to a bowl and season with salt to taste. Remove soup from heat. Add lime juice and zest. Season with salt and pepper to taste. Ladle into bowls. Top with pumpkin seeds.

Health Benefits of Winter Squash

Act as natural anti-inflammatory. Contain high dose of key nutrients for pregnant women. Squash puree can be used as an effective hydrating and toning mask for chapped winter skin.

37. Chili Made Easy

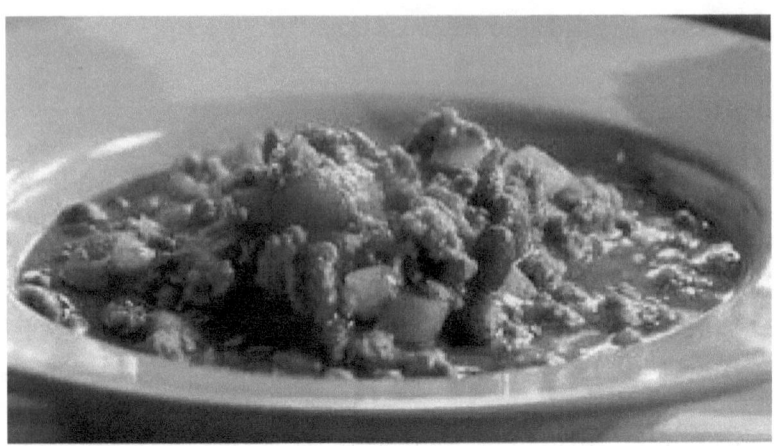

This quick chili is hearty and delicious. It's also packed with multiple servings of veggies.

Ingredients

- ☐ 1 lbs. Ground Beef (80% lean)
- ☐ 1 Red Bell Pepper (diced)
- ☐ 1 Green Bell Pepper (diced)
- ☐ 1 Onion (chopped)
- ☐ 1 (32oz.) can Whole Tomatoes (chopped)
- ☐ 3 Tbsps. Olive Oil
- ☐ 1 Tbsp. Molasses
- ☐ 1 Tbsp. Chili Powder
- ¾ tsp Cinnamon

- Salt & Pepper to taste

- 1 tsp Unsweetened Cocoa Powder

- Sour Cream

Method

1. Heat oil in a deep pan over medium-high heat. Add onion. Cook until golden (about 8 minutes). Add bell peppers. Cook 6 minutes. Add cocoa, chili powder, salt, pepper, and cinnamon. Cook 1 minute, stirring constantly.

2. Add beef. Cook until no longer pink. Stir to break up lumps. Add molasses and tomatoes with juice. Simmer until thickened (about 5-8 minutes).

Health Benefits of Bell Peppers

Help increase libido. Maintains collagen and helps reduce wrinkles. Speed up metabolism.

38. Clam Chowder

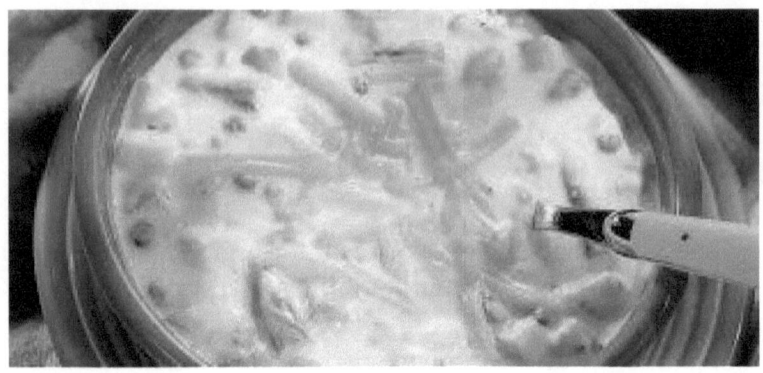

Create a rich and satisfying clam chowder quickly with this ingenious recipe.

Ingredients

- ½ lbs. Bacon (chopped)
- 2 lbs. Potatoes (peeled, diced)
- 2 (6.5oz.) cans Chopped Clams
- 2 (8oz.) bottles Clam Juice
- 1 cup Water
- 1 cup Half & Half
- 2 Carrots (chopped)
- 3 stalks Celery (chopped)
- 1 Onion (chopped)
- 1 tsp Garlic Powder

- ¼ cup Fresh Parsley (chopped)

Method

1. In a large pan over medium heat, cook bacon until light brown. Leave about 2 tablespoons of fat. Drain the rest. Add carrots, onion, celery, and garlic powder. Cook 5 minutes.

2. Add clam juice, water, juice from the canned clams, and potatoes. Bring to a boil. Reduce heat and simmer 20 minutes (uncovered). Add half and half and clams. Simmer 5 minutes. Season with salt and pepper to taste. Sprinkle with parsley. Serve.

Health Benefits of Clams

Just 4 oz. of clams contain about 17x your daily B12 requirements. B12 helps protect brain health and maintains healthy red blood cells. Clams also boast a full supply of iron.

39. Simplified Cioppino

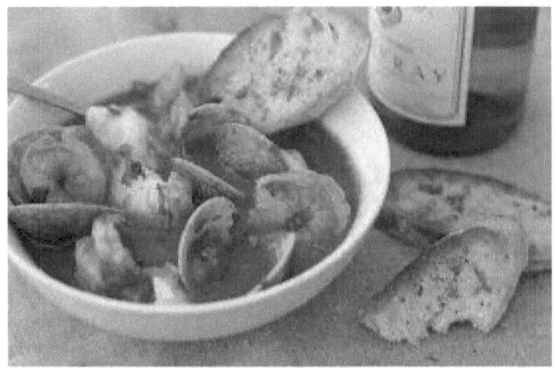

This quick and easy seafood stew will have you dreaming of the seaside.

Ingredients

- ☐ 1 lbs. White Fish Fillets (skinless, cubed)
- ☐ 1 lbs. Mussels
- ☐ 1 (8oz.) bottle Clam Juice
- ☐ 1 cup Red Wine
- • 1 ½ cups Water
- ☐ 1 (28oz.) can Crushed Tomatoes
- ☐ 1 bulb Fennel (in wedges)
- ☐ 1 Onion (quartered)
- ☐ 3 cloves Garlic (crushed)
- ☐ 3 Tbsps. Olive Oil

- 1 ½ tsp Thyme

- 1 tsp Crushed Red Pepper Flakes

- 2 Bay Leaves

Method

1. In a food processor, coarsely chop onion, fennel, and garlic. Heat oil in a large pot on medium-high heat. Stir in chopped onion mixture. Add thyme, salt, pepper, crushed red pepper flakes, and bay leaves. Cover and cook 4 minutes.

2. Add tomatoes with juice. Add water, wine, and clam juice. Bring to a boil. Cover and cook 20 minutes. Stir in seafood. Cook 4-6 minutes, uncovered (until mussels open and fish is just cooked through. Discard bay leaves.

Health Benefits of Mussels

High in depression-fighting selenium. 1 cup contains 18 grams of protein. High in vitamin A which is needed for your eyes, skin, hair, teeth, and nails.

40. Veggie & Almond Couscous

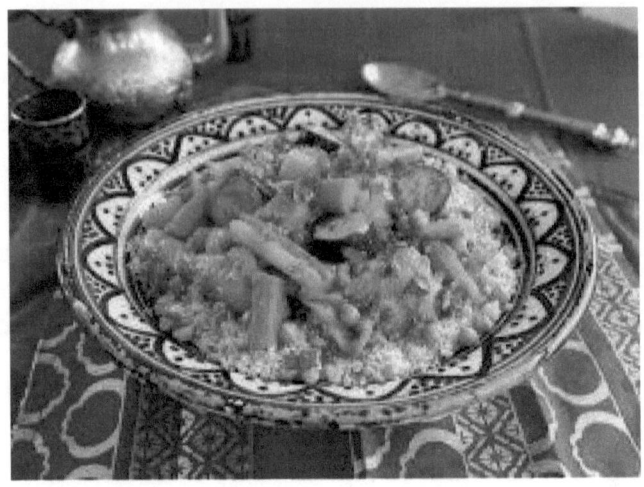

Prepare this deliciously light but satisfying meal in under 30 minutes.

Ingredients

- 1/3 cup Sliced Almonds
- 3 cups Mixed Veggies (chopped)
- 1 cup Dry White Wine
- ¾ cup Vegetable Broth
- 1/3 cup Golden Raisins
- 1 (7oz.) box Couscous and Lentil Mix
- 1 Tbsp. Olive Oil
- 1 ½ tsp Cumin
- 1 ½ tsp Coriander

Method

1. Cook almonds in a pan over medium heat until lightly golden (about 4 minutes). Stir often. Transfer to a bowl. Add oil to the same pan. Increase heat to medium-high. Add veggies, coriander, and cumin. Cook 3 minutes. Add raisins and wine. Boil 3 minutes. Add broth. Cover halfway and simmer 6 minutes.

2. Season with salt and pepper to taste. Prepare couscous according to instructions on box. Place the couscous in a mound on a platter. Spoon the veggies and broth over the top. Sprinkle with almonds.

Health Benefits of Almonds

Help lower cholesterol. High in skin-nourishing vitamin E. High bone-strengthening phosphorus.

41. Paella

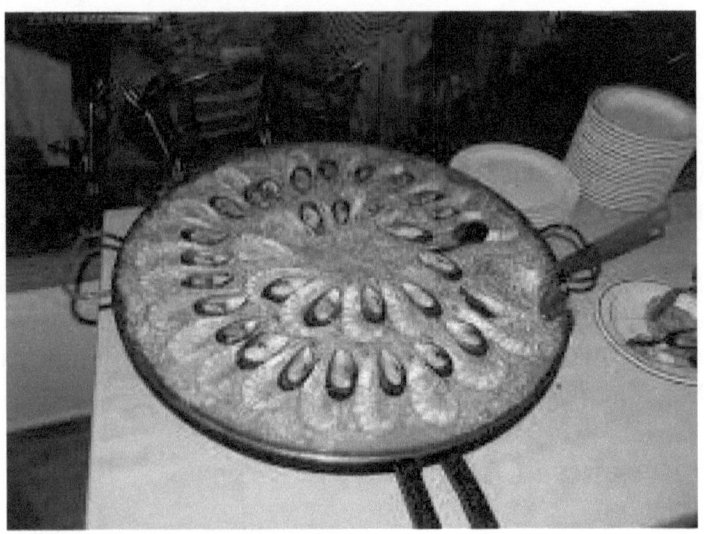

This quick paella with chorizo and saffron rice is sure to be a crowd-pleaser.

Ingredients

- ¾ lbs. Chorizo (chopped)
- 1 lbs. Saffron Rice
- 1 (9oz.) package Frozen Artichoke Hearts
- 1 lbs. Jumbo Shrimp (peeled)
- 2 cups Chicken Broth (or Wine)
- 1 cup Frozen Peas
- 1 (8oz.) jar Roasted Red Peppers (drained, sliced)
- 4 Tbsps. Olive Oil

Method

1. Brown the chorizo in a pan. Add rice, peppers, artichoke hearts, 2 cups water, and broth (or wine). Bring to a boil.

2. Reduce heat and simmer with the lid on until most of the liquid is absorbed (about 20 minutes). Add peas and shrimp. Cover and cook 5-7 minutes.

Health Benefits of Peas

High in fiber and protein which helps you control appetite and lose weight. A cup of peas per day can dramatically lower your risk for cancer. Protects your body from age-related degradation.

42. Tomato Bouillabaisse

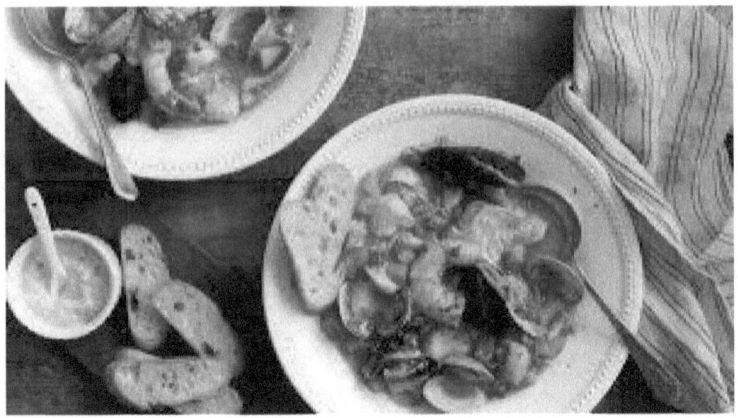

You may not be able to pronounce it but that won't stop you from coming back for a second helping of this seafood dish.

Ingredients

- ☐ 3 lbs. Mixed Shellfish (scrubbed)
- ☐ 4 cups Cherry Tomatoes
- ½ cup Fresh Basil Leaves
- ¼ cup Mayonnaise
- ¼ cup Dry White Wine
- ☐ 1 bulb Fennel (trimmed, halved, sliced)
- ☐ 2 Anchovy Fillets in Oil (drained)
- ☐ 4 cloves Garlic
- ☐ 1 (8oz.) bottle Clam Juice

- 5 Tbsps. Olive Oil

- 1 Tbsp. Fresh Lemon Juice

- Salt & Pepper to taste

- Crusty Bread (sliced)

Method

1. Mince 2 garlic cloves. Pour into a blender. Add mayonnaise, basil, 3 tablespoons oil, lemon juice, and anchovies. Puree until smooth. Transfer to a small bowl. Cover and chill.

2. Heat 2 tablespoons oil in a large pot on medium-high heat. Add tomatoes and fennel. Season with salt and pepper to taste. Cook until tomatoes burst (about 10 minutes). Stir occasionally.

3. Slice 2 garlic cloves thinly. Add to pot. Cook about 1 minute. Pour in the wine. Cook 1 minute, stirring constantly. Add 4 cups water and clam juice. Bring to a boil. Add shellfish, cover and cook until shellfish open (about 3 minutes). Spread the basil-mayonnaise mixture on slices of crusty bread and serve alongside.

Health Benefits of Shellfish

Contains as much protein as red meat but in a more easily digestible form. Contains more omega-3s than tuna. Shellfish are also high in potassium and other key minerals.

43. Orange Chicken Stir Fry

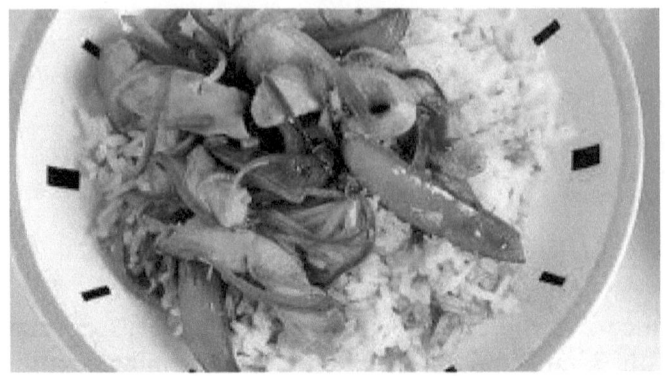

Say goodbye to congealed fast food orange chicken and hello to this quick and easy stir fry.

Ingredients

- 1 ½ cups Jasmine Rice
- 1 ½ lbs. Chicken Cutlets (cut into strips)
- ¾ cups Orange Juice
- ☐ 1 (8oz.) package String-less Snap Peas
- ☐ 1 Red Onion (halved, sliced)
- ☐ 3 Tbsps. Soy Sauce
- ☐ 2 Tbsps. Olive Oil
- ☐ 1 Tbsp. Corn Starch
- ☐ 2 tsp Orange Zest
- ☐ 1 tsp Crushed Red Pepper Flakes

Method

1. In a large pot bring rice and 3 cups water to a boil. Reduce heat, cover, and simmer until liquid is absorbed. In a bowl, whisk together cornstarch, soy sauce, and orange juice. Mix in zest. Heat oil in a large pan over high heat. Add crushed red pepper flakes and onion. Fry 30 seconds.

2. Sprinkle salt and pepper over the chicken. Add chicken to pan and cook 4 minutes. Add snap peas and juice mixture to pan. Toss until sauce boils and thickens (about 2 minutes). Season with salt and pepper to taste. Serve over rice.

Health Benefits of Snap Peas

High in folic acid. High in vitamin C. High in B vitamins.

44. Sausage & Kale Fettuccine

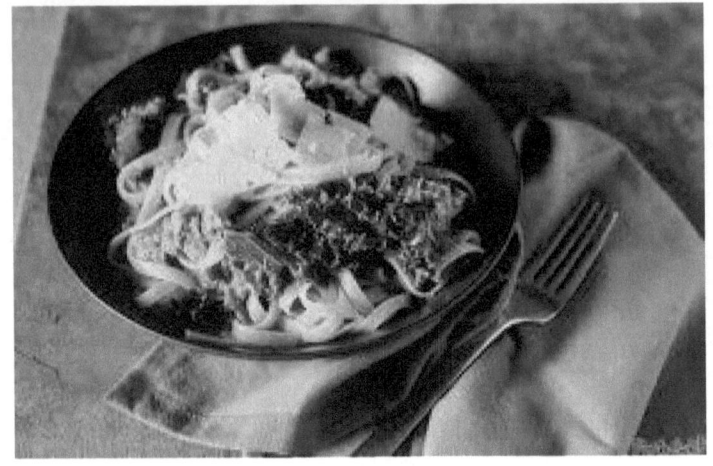

Get your daily serving of kale with this deliciously simple fettuccine.

Ingredients

- ☐ 1 lbs. Pork or Turkey Sausage (casings removed, crumbled)
- ½ lbs. Kale (chopped)
- ½ lbs. Fettuccine
- ☐ 2/3 cup Chicken Broth
- ½ cup Pecorino Romano (grated)
- ☐ 3 Tbsps. Olive Oil

Method

1. Heat oil in a large pan over high heat. Brown sausage, stirring to break apart lumps. Blanch kale in a pot of boiling salted water for 5 minutes. Remove kale and drain.

2. Reserve salted water and return it to boiling. Add fettuccine. Cook until slightly undercooked. Reserve 1 cup of salted water and drain pasta.

3. While pasta is cooking, add kale to the pan with sausage. Cook 5 minutes, stirring often. Stir in broth. Add pasta and ½ cup reserved salted water. Toss to combine. Stir in cheese with the remaining ½ cup salted water.

Health Benefits of Kale

High in fiber. High in iron. High in vitamin K.

45. Mushroom & Sausage Lasagna

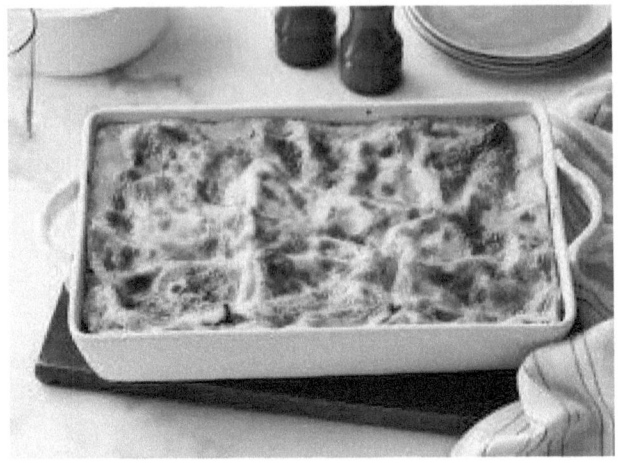

Lasagna just got easier with this quick and scrumptious recipe.

Ingredients

- ☐ 1 (9oz.) package No-Cook Lasagna Noodles
- ☐ 1 lbs. Italian Sausage (casings removed)
- ☐ 1 lbs. Mushrooms (sliced)
- ☐ 1 (15oz.) package Ricotta
- ☐ 2 cups Mozzarella (grated)
- ☐ 2 cups Cheddar (grated)
- ☐ 4 2/3 cups Marinara Sauce
- ☐ 1 cup Dry Red Wine
- ☐ 2 cups Onion (chopped)

- 3 cloves Garlic (crushed)

- 2 Tbsps. Herb Blend (your preference)

- 2 Tbsps. Olive Oil

Method

1. Preheat oven to 400°F. Heat oil in a large pot on high heat. Add onion, mushroom, and herb blend. Cook 6 minutes. Add sausage. Cook 5 minutes, stirring to break apart chunks. Stir in garlic. Cook 1 minute.

2. Stir in wine. Cook until liquid is reduced by half (about 2-3 minutes). Set aside. Spread 2/3 cup marinara over bottom of a baking dish. Place a layer of noodles on top of the sauce. Spread 1 cup marinara over the noodles.

3. Spread 1/3 of the ricotta on top. Then spread 1 cup cheese over that. Spoon 1/3 of sausage mixture over the cheese. Repeat this process 2 more times with the remaining ingredients. Cover with foil but avoid letting the chees touch the foil. Bake 45 minutes. Remove foil. Bake an additional 10 minutes (or until bubbly and browned). Let cool 15 minutes.

Health Benefits of Mushrooms

Natural dietary source of vitamin D. High in iron. Helps boost immune system.

46. Sautéed Ham & Brussels Sprouts

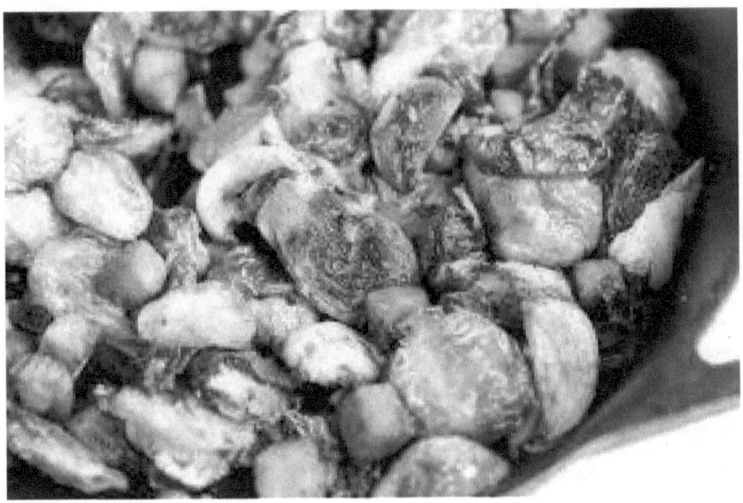

This richly flavored Brussels sprouts dish makes a perfect side to a creamy pasta or grilled fish.

Ingredients

- ☐ 2 lbs. Brussels Sprouts (roots trimmed)
- ☐ 6 oz. Smoked Ham (chopped)
- ☐ 2/3 cup Chicken Broth
- • ½ cup Toasted Pecans (chopped)
- ☐ 1 clove Garlic (minced)
- ☐ 3 Tbsps. Olive Oil
- ☐ 2 Tbsps. Butter
- ☐ Salt to taste

Method

1. Shred Brussels sprouts in a food processor. Cover and chill. Heat butter and oil in a large pan over medium heat. Add ham. Cook 3 minutes (or until golden). Stir in garlic. Cook 30 seconds.

2. Add broth and chilled Brussels sprouts. Cook until crisp and tender (about 3-5 minutes). Season with salt and pepper to taste. Transfer to a serving bowl. Sprinkle with pecans.

Health Benefits of Brussels Sprouts

Helps lower cholesterol. Helps protect DNA from damage. Acts as natural anti-inflammatory.

47. Salmon in Blueberry Sauce

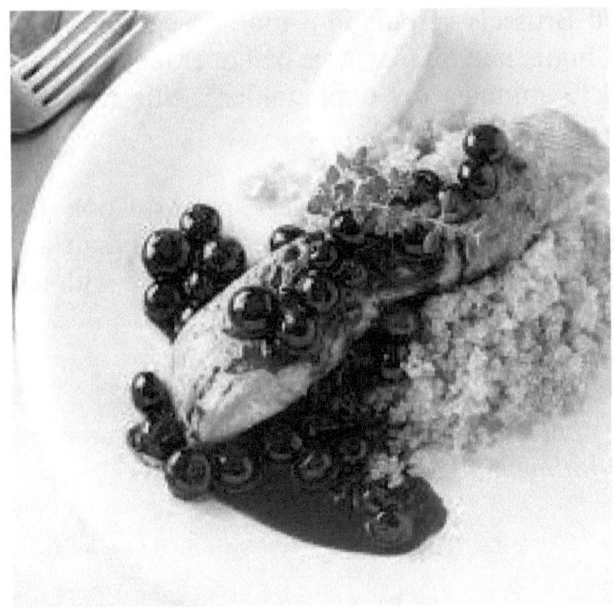

Effortlessly balance sweet and savory in this beautiful salmon dish.

Ingredients

- 4 (7oz.) Salmon Fillets (with skin)
- 1 cup Blueberries
- ¼ cup Water
- ¾ cup Shallots (sliced)
- 1 clove Garlic (sliced)
- 3 Tbsps. Fresh Mint (chopped)
- 1 Tbsp. Balsamic Vinegar

- 1 Tbsp. Olive Oil
- 1 tsp Thyme
- ½ tsp Allspice
- Salt to taste

Method

1. Heat 1 tablespoon oil in a large pan on medium heat. Add shallots. Cook 5 minutes. Add garlic, thyme, allspice, and salt. Cook 30 seconds, stirring constantly. Add blueberries, vinegar, and ¼ cup water. Blend well. Stir and mash berries until sauce thickens (about 3-4 minutes). Season with pepper to taste. Set aside.

2. Lightly oil the grill rack. Prepare barbecue for medium-high heat. Lightly brush both sides of the salmon with oil. Sprinkle with thyme, allspice, salt, and pepper.

3. Grill salmon 4-5 minutes on each side. Transfer to plates. Stir 2 tablespoons of the fresh mint into the blueberry sauce. Spoon over the salmon. Sprinkle remaining mint over the tops of each fillet.

Health Benefits of Blueberries

Ranked 1st on the list of foods with most antioxidants. Helps get rid of belly fat. Helps treat symptoms of urinary tract infections.

48. Chicken Masala

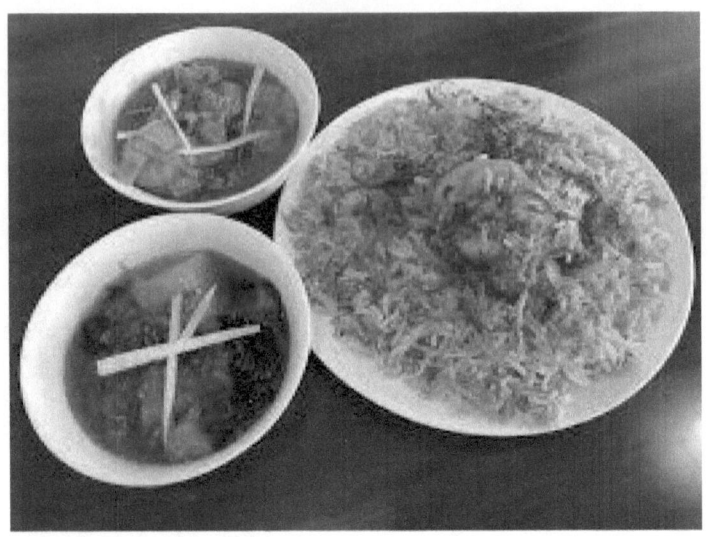

This rich and creamy marinade makes for a juicy and delicious dinner.

Ingredients

- 4 ½ lbs. Whole Chicken (backbone removed, cut into 8 pieces)
- 2 Onions (sliced)
- 1 cup Plain Greek Yogurt
- ¼ cup Cilantro
- 1 clove Garlic (crushed)
- 3 Tbsps. Olive Oil
- 1 Tbsp. Garam Masala
- Salt to taste

Method

1. In a baking dish, combine yogurt, olive oil, garlic, cilantro, and garam masala. Add chicken pieces. Coat all sides. Cover with plastic wrap and refrigerate at least 2 hours (up to 1 day). Preheat oven to 400°F.

2. Arrange onions in a large baking dish to form a bed for the chicken. Place chicken pieces on top of onions. Make sure none of the pieces are touching. Cook 1 hour or until chicken is cooked through. Drizzle pan juices over chicken before serving.

Health Benefits of Greek Yogurt

Full of key probiotics that help improve digestion and immune system. Amino acids help heal sore muscles after a workout. High calcium content helps lower cortisol levels (a stress hormone that causes you to store belly fat).

49. Lamb Provencal

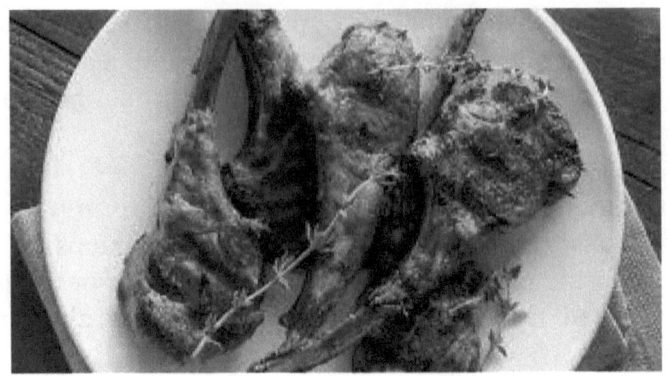

This is an effortlessly exquisite lamb dish with just the right balance of herbs and seasoning.

Ingredients

- ☐ 1 (6-7 lbs.) Leg of Lamb (bone in, trimmed, tied)
- ½ cup Dijon Mustard
- ☐ 3 lbs. Tomatoes (diced)
- ½ cup Olive Oil
- ½ cup Honey
- ☐ 1 Onion (sliced)
- ☐ 9 cloves Garlic (chopped)
- ☐ 4 sprigs Thyme
- ☐ 2 sprigs Rosemary
- ☐ 1 Tbsp. Balsamic Vinegar

- 1 Tbsp. Dried Rosemary

- Salt & Pepper to taste

Method

1. Preheat oven to 450°F. Place leg of lamb on a large roasting pan (fat side up). Pat dry with paper towels. In a food processor, pulse together mustard, 1 tablespoon garlic, rosemary, balsamic vinegar, salt, and pepper. Spread garlic-vinegar mixture over the lamb.

2. In a bowl, toss together tomatoes, olive oil, onion, ¼ cup honey, and remaining garlic. Pour the tomato mixture around the lamb. Tuck in the thyme and rosemary sprigs. Drizzle the remaining ¼ cup honey over the lamb. Roast 20 minutes.

3. Reduce heat to 350°F and roast for 1 hour or until meat thermometer reds 130°-135°F. Place lamb on a cutting board. Cover with foil. Let rest 15 minutes. Return tomatoes to oven to stay warm. Slice lamb. Arrange on plates. Top with tomatoes and pan juices.

Health Benefits of Lamb

High in protein High in vitamin BHigh in iron.

50. Glazed Pork Chops

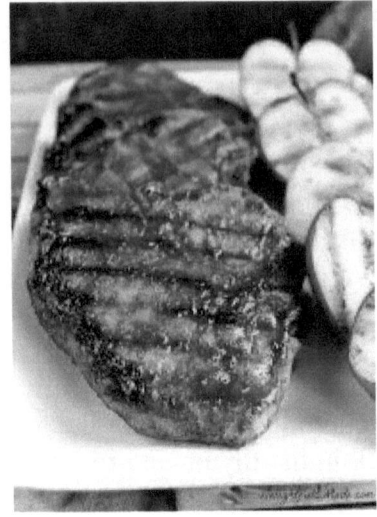

This glazed pork chops recipe comes with a wonderfully simple veggie side dish to create a complete dinner.

Ingredients

- ☐ 4 Pork Chops
- • ¾ cup Balsamic Vinegar
- ☐ 1 head Endive (quartered)
- ☐ 1 head Radicchio (quartered)
- ☐ 3 Tbsps. Olive Oil
- ☐ 3 Tbsps. Salt
- ☐ 1 Tbsp. Butter
- • 1 ½ Tbsps. Sugar

Method

1. Prepare barbecue at medium-high heat. In a baking dish, combine 1 ½ cups water, salt, and sugar. Add pork chops. Brine 20 minutes turning occasionally. Arrange endive and radicchio on a baking sheet. Brush with oil. Sprinkle with salt and pepper.

2. In a small pan, boil vinegar for 5 minutes (or until reduced to ¼ cup. Whisk in butter. Season with salt and pepper. Remove pork chops from brine. Pat dry. Brush with oil and sprinkle with pepper.

3. Grill pork, endives, and radicchio until vegetables are softened and meat thermometer reads 150°F (about 2-3 minutes for the veggies and 7-8 per side for the pork). Transfer pork and veggies to plates. Drizzle with butter vinegar glaze.

Health Benefits of Radicchio

Acts as a natural pain reliever. Improves digestion. Improves cognitive function.

Conclusion

Food is one of the basic necessities of living. In the mundane series of things, food is one of the things that excites us, influences us and brings about a change in our outward as well as internal persona. Cultures are defined and remembered by the food they eat, the recipes they make, the spices they incorporate.

This recipe book has combined food from different cultures ranging from Moroccon to Arabic to Chinese, taking us through the world. In a whirlwind of our busy lives, we can find solace of enjoying different cultures in the very comforts of our own home.

These easy to cook recipes, ranging from poultry to vegetables to seafood will bring about a healthy and flavorful change. This recipe book seeks to provide you with a complete four course meal option including a refreshing drink to complete the orgasmic experience! Moreover, all these recipes serve as your savior and all those metabolic illnesses which make life shorter and tiresome!

We hope that this recipe book brings about a constructive change in your life. And you enjoy preparing these wonderful recipes with those you love and want to spend a long and healthy life with.

Final Words

I would like to thank you for downloading my book and I hope I have been able to help you and educate you about something new.

If you have enjoyed this book and would like to share your positive thoughts, could you please take 30 seconds of your time to go back and give me a review on my Amazon book page!

I greatly appreciate seeing these reviews because it helps me share my hard work!

Again, thank you and I wish you all the best with your cooking journey!

Last Chance to Get YOUR Bonus!

FOR A LIMITED TIME ONLY – Get Olivia's best-selling book *"The #1 Cookbook: Over 170+ of the Most Popular Recipes Across 7 Different Cuisines!"* absolutely FREE!

Readers have absolutely loved this book because of the wide variety of recipes. It is highly recommended you check these recipes out and see what you can add to your home menu!

Once again, as a big thank-you for downloading this book, I'd like to offer it to you *100% FREE for a LIMITED TIME ONLY!*

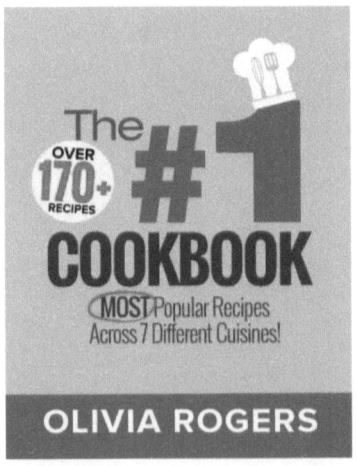

Get your free copy at:

TheMenuAtHome.com/Bonus

Disclaimer

This book and related site provides recipe and food advice in an informative and educational manner only, with information that is general in nature and that is not specific to you, the reader. The contents of this book and related site are intended to assist you and other readers in your personal efforts. Consult your physician or nutritionist regarding the applicability of any information provided in our information to you.

Nothing in this book should be construed as personal advice or diagnosis, and must not be used in this manner. The information provided about conditions is general in nature. This information does not cover all possible uses, actions, precautions, side-effects, or interactions of medicines, or medical procedures. The information in this site should not be considered as complete and does not cover all diseases, ailments, physical conditions, or their treatment.

No Warranties: The authors and publishers don't guarantee or warrant the quality, accuracy, completeness, timeliness, appropriateness or suitability of the information in this book, or of any product or services referenced by this site.

The information in this site is provided on an "as is" basis and the authors and publishers make no representations or warranties of any kind with respect to this information. This site may contain inaccuracies, typographical errors, or other errors.

Liability Disclaimer: The publishers, authors, and other parties involved in the creation, production, provision of information, or delivery of this site specifically disclaim any responsibility, and shall not be held liable for any damages, claims, injuries, losses, liabilities, costs, or obligations including any direct, indirect, special, incidental, or consequences damages (collectively known as "Damages") whatsoever and howsoever caused, arising out of, or in connection with the use or misuse of the site and the information contained within it, whether such Damages arise in contract, tort, negligence, equity, statute law, or by way of other legal theory.

www.ingramcontent.com/pod-product-compliance
Lightning Source LLC
Chambersburg PA
CBHW031128080526
44587CB00011B/1150